The Essential Tantra

I am circling around God, around the ancient tower,
and I have been circling for a thousand years,
and I still don't know if I am a falcon, or a storm,
or a great song.

—Rainer Maria Rilke

Also by Kenneth Ray Stubbs, Ph.D.

Erotic Massage
Secret Sexual Positions
Romantic Interludes: A Sensuous Lovers Guide
The Clitoral Kiss: A Fun Guide to Oral Sex, Oral Massage,
and Other Oral Delights
Male Erotic Massage: A Guide to Sex and Spirit
Women of the Light: The New Sacred Prostitute
(editor, contributor)
Tantric Massage Video

THE ESSENTIAL TANTRA

A Modern Guide
to Sacred Sexuality

Kenneth Ray Stubbs, Ph.D.

**Illustrated by
Kyle Spencer and Richard Stodart**

Jeremy P. Tarcher/Putnam
a member of Penguin Putnam Inc.
New York

Most Tarcher/Putnam books are available at special quantity discounts for bulk purchase for sales promotions, premiums, fund-raising, and educational needs. Special books or book excerpts also can be created to fit specific needs. For details, write Putnam Special Markets, 375 Hudson Street, New York, NY 10014.

A Word of Caution

The purpose of this book is to educate. It is not intended to give medical or psychological therapy. Whenever there is concern about physical or emotional illness, a qualified professional should be consulted.

All the sexual positions, rituals, and activities in this book are not for every body. Some of the positions were accomplished only after years of yogic practice.

Because of the litigation-happy times in which we live, here is the necessary legal disclaimer:

The author, illustrator, and publisher shall have neither liability nor responsibility to any person or entity with respect to any loss, damage, injury, or ailment caused or alleged to be caused directly or indirectly by the information or lack of information in this book.

So take responsibility for your own health. Please don't get stuck in a position you can't get out of.

Jeremy P. Tarcher/Putnam
A member of
Penguin Putnam Inc.
375 Hudson Street
New York, NY 10014
www.penguinputnam.com

First Jeremy P. Tarcher edition 1999
Originally published by Secret Garden, Larkspur, California
Tantric Massage was originally published as *Erotic Massage*
by Jeremy P. Tarcher/Putnam in 1998
Copyright © 1989, 1993 by Kenneth Ray Stubbs, Ph.D.
Illustrations by Kyle Spencer. Based on photography by Ellen Gunther.
Chapter Heading Artwork by Richard Stodart.
Sensual Ceremony text copyright © 1993 by Kenneth Ray Stubbs, Ph.D.
Illustrations copyright © 1993 by Richard Stodart.
Sacred Orgasms copyright © 1992 by Kenneth Ray Stubbs, Ph.D.
Illustrations copyright © 1999 by Richard Stodart.

Library of Congress Cataloging-in-Publication Data

Stubbs, Kenneth Ray.
The essential tantra : a modern guide to sacred sexuality / by Kenneth Ray Stubbs;
illustrated by Kyle Spencer and Richard Stodart.
p.   cm.
ISBN 1-58542-014-X
1. Sex instruction.   I. Title.
HQ31.S989   1999   99-052424
613.9'6—dc21

Printed in the United States of America

1   3   5   7   9   10   8   6   4   2

This book is printed on acid-free paper. ∞

The Essential Tantra

Acceptance
        is a central teaching
        in tantric traditions
Embracing the whole,
        we transcend
                the world of duality

Today in the West
        tantra
                has often come to mean
        sacred sex, spiritual sexuality, sexual spirituality
It is in this context
        that I use
tantric massage:
        touching
                the sexual and spiritual dimensions
                        within each of us
                —with full acceptance
                —embracing an apparent duality

Volume I - *Tantric Massage*
        presents specific, practical
                massage techniques
        for the *whole* body

Volume II - *Sensual Ceremony*
        brings to massage and other pleasuring experiences
        the context of ceremony,
                a meditation
                        in the realm of the senses

Volume III - *Sacred Orgasms*
        proposes the encompassing paradigm of the trilogy:
                the extent to which
                        we deny our spirituality
                        we limit our sexuality
                the extent to which
                        we judge our sexuality
                        we limit our spirituality
        Here, orgasm
                is the teacher

CONTENTS

SENSUAL CEREMONY

SACRED ORGASMS

AFTERWORD:
SACRED SEXUAL POSITIONS

PREFACE

This book began twenty years ago as a manuscript that attracted no publishers. So I decided to modify the text into several smaller books and publish them myself.

After seeing that the books had been well received, the editors at Tarcher/Putnam agreed with my proposal to bring three of the books out as a single volume. Presented together in one source, the writings and illustrations support a much deeper understanding of the essential role our sexuality can serve on a spiritual path.

Tantric Massage, along with its earlier edition, *Erotic Massage,* was the first book to illustrate genital massage. (There is far more censorship and *de facto* censorship than most people realize.) Intended for present and potential sexual partners, this book focuses on long, flowing strokes to nurture the whole being. The thorough step-by-step massage is gentle rather than athletic and does not require the giver to be particularly muscular.

Sensual Ceremony, exactly as the name describes, brings a meditative, ceremonial context to the sensual and sexual, without requiring a meditation background. Bathing, feeding, massaging, guided inner journeys for modern Western lovers—these are all to deepen intimacy and a sense of communion.

Sacred Orgasms is a paradigm with orgasm at the center of the sacred circle. This greatly revised edition presents teachings and a specific set of meditations that a group of five masterful beings communicated to me with the intent that the knowledge be included in this book.

An art section on sexual positions follows that teaches about the heart as much as about sex.

In these quite diverse yet very connected writings, I have shared my realization that the sensual and the sexual, rather than being obstacles on the spiritual path, are actually one with the sacred. I encourage you to explore the many practical techniques and meditations within to discover for yourself this ancient understanding.

INTRODUCTION TO
THE ESSENTIAL TANTRA

In tantra, everything is sacred. And there are no sacred cows.

Tantra has never been a chosen path for me. It's just a path on which I've continued finding my feet.

Over twenty-five years ago, a teacher of sorts began to communicate with me, sort of.

After completing massage school in San Francisco, I began to massage professionally. Massaging men and women, I often would have sexual feelings, not necessarily intense, but still obviously sexual.

These were days of high testosterone levels when I would sit down to meditate and end up masturbating. Quieting my breath and my mind in meditation, I would only become more aware of how horny I really was. Moreover, since massage had evolved into a form of meditation for me, I seemed to be keenly aware of my sexual feelings when giving a massage.

Basically, two main options seemed available: I could suppress and deny my sexual feelings in massage, or I could embrace them consciously. Exploring the latter, I decided to offer classes in erotic massage. Providing sexual entertainment to the public did not appeal to me personally. The thought of teaching anyone nurturing touch and subtle lovemaking in a context of trust, however, felt deeply meaningful.

I began arrangements for giving a weekend couples workshop at a massage and yoga center. Preparing the brochure with some friends, I talked about teaching foot bathing and facial massage to relax the couples and to bring a nurturing ambience to sexual touch. Genital massage would be included. Orgasm or intercourse would not be the goal, just pleasure for the *whole* body and being.

Genital massage was something absolutely forbidden in massage school and not illustrated in any massage book at that time. Yet, we all knew that sexual partners often explore creative adaptations in the bedroom once they learn some general massage strokes.

While discussing these ideas and preparing the brochure with my friends, I casually mentioned that this would actually be a modern tantra workshop. Precisely the moment I said the word *tantra*, a clearly audible ringing occurred just exterior to my right ear for about one to two seconds.

The first such ringing had occurred only a few weeks earlier while attending a metaphysical class on astral projection. The teacher would often lead us in a guided imagery meditation to visit with our *spirit companions*, as she called them. Usually nothing seemed to happen for me, no clear images, no messages, nothing but a nice nap.

Then one evening in class, while we were moving around during a break, out of the blue I heard my first clear ringing. When I told my teacher, she suggested the ringing might be a spirit companion coming close to my energetic field to communicate. After a few more ringings in the next months, I began a journal of the ringings. There were no voices, words, or images. So I wrote what was happening or what I was thinking or saying at the moment of the ringing, treating the sound as an indication to pay close attention to what was occurring.

A predominant pattern became apparent over several years: The ringing occurred most often when I was thinking or talking about tantra.

Tantra is an Eastern spiritual philosophy. Initially coming to us from approximately third and fourth century C.E. India, this experiential examination of existence evolved from many roots in antiquity and was adapted and modified in a myriad of subcultures and religions. Both India and Tibet, both Hinduism and Buddhism, have many variants of tantra. Chinese Taoism and tantra have many resemblances. Indeed, in their popular evolutions in the modern West, these two philosophical systems are often mingled into a single framework.

Tantra, a Sanskrit word, is similar to our concept of weaving. "The web of life" and "the interconnectedness of all that is" are useful connotations for understanding tantra as a philosophy. My simplified version is "embracing all" or "acceptance of all."

In general, this philosophy emphasizes practical, experiential approaches. Central to the many variations is this teaching: Rather than being obstacles, our sensory experiences can be a path to spiritual wholeness, to at-one-ment.

In stark contrast to beliefs of atonement, so dearly held in our modern Western religions, tantra teaches neither the flesh as inherently evil nor the spirit as inherently good.

In tantra, it is the body and the senses that provide vehicles for us to go beyond the duality of evil and good. Learning to perceive and transform subtle energies, we can rediscover essence, which is the sacred connection of everything.

A story about the three main schools of thought in Buddhism conveys the meaning of *transformation*.

A practitioner of one school is walking down the path of life. Upon seeing a poisonous plant in the middle of the path, the practitioner turns around to follow another route.

A practitioner of the second school is walking down the same path and also sees the poisonous plant. Instead of turning back in the opposite direction, this practitioner cautiously detours slightly around the poisonous plant, sort of like letting a sleeping dog lie, and continues on down the path.

A practitioner of the third school, also on the same path, upon seeing the plant says, "Yes, now I can learn about this poison." He or she then sits down and begins to consume the plant.

Applying powerful transformational skills gained over many years of meditation, the practitioner is able to become at-one with the essence of the plant and the poison. And the poison is no longer poisonous, for the poison and the practitioner are no longer different or opposite. They are no longer in disharmony.

Here we have transformed our emotions into a willingness to connect with what we are avoiding (the poison). We have also transformed our emotions into a willingness to let go of what we are grasping (continued life).

Moreover, we have transformed ourselves so we have the ability to resonate our energies in harmony with the essence of others' energies. Even potentially harmful energies (here the poisonous chemical) cease being harmful because with conscious intent we are able to vibrate our energies in the same patterns as the poison's. Energetically, we become the same as the poison.

Ultimately, these are what the transformation teachings are about in tantric philosophy.

This third school of thought is known as Vajrayana Buddhism, or Tantric Buddhism, and comes principally from Tibet. While an oversimplification of the different main schools of Buddhism, the story exemplifies the heart of tantric philosophy: Embracing all, tantra goes beyond graspings and avoidances—our sacred cows—into essence. In the river of essence, there are no attachments, only energy flowing.

My personal journey into my body and the senses took me to experiences and understandings I never anticipated while growing up as a fundamentalist Christian.

Massage brought me back to my body after many years in academia. I began to listen with my hands. I began to express more of my heart through my touch. All of the emotions, not just sexual feelings, became more evident in others and myself. Many physical pleasures reawoke.

Studying and meditating with a Tibetan Buddhist lama, my ability to experience the subtle energies deepened. My mindfulness/awareness/consciousness became more focused. Meditating after doing specific movements and specific postures, I learned how to more keenly observe my mind and sensations in my physical and subtle energy bodies. In meditative practice, the lama would remind us to bring our conscious awareness to the most intense sensation and just observe. Regardless if the sensation be pleasurable, painful, or neutral, let go of analyzing and simply experience the sensation fully. Be at-one with the sensation.

Though the Tibetan lama was definitely from a Tantric Buddhist lineage, he spoke about sex only once in my presence. My experience of Eastern sexual practices would come much more from a Chinese Taoist teacher. In this tradition, men are advised, as a means to conserve energy, to limit or refrain from ejaculating. For me, riding a long sexual wave without orgasming or attempting to orgasm without ejaculation became a major sexual focus for several years. Exploring my attachment to an ejaculatory orgasm brought many insights and many liberations.

Because of my academic background and what I taught in my erotic massage workshops, I was invited to teach human sexuality graduate students a fifty-hour course in massage and body approaches in sex therapy and counseling. The more I taught, the more I found there was to learn from the blossoming field of scientific Western sexology.

Then one day East met West. Suddenly I realized that what I was learning about meditation from the Tibetan lama and what Masters and Johnson were doing in their highly effective sex therapy techniques known as sensate focus are fundamentally the same.

The Masters and Johnson sensate focus exercises are incredibly simple and yet often profound for those of us stuck in our heads or stuck in the belief that sex and the flesh are innately sinful.

Both partners are nude. One touches the other, the receiver simply feeling the sensation and giving feedback regarding the desirability of the sensation. In these exercises, intercourse is excluded. In addition, initially the male and female genitals and the female breasts are excluded in the touching. The underlying objective in these sensate focus exercises is the same as in many forms of meditation: Be here now. Consciously focusing our awareness on any sensation, whether it be our breath or the touch of a beloved, can bring us into the present moment.

To the extent we approach lovemaking as a moment-to-moment unfoldment, many sexual dysfunctions disappear. Whatever loving and/or erotic connection already exists can intensify. Many joys can awaken.

When we approach life as a moment-to-moment unfoldment, many of our attachments become unbound. William Blake said it best:

> He who binds himself to a joy
> Doth the winged life destroy;
> But he who kisses the joy as it flies
> Lives in eternity's sunrise

As I taught and studied more about sexuality and spirituality in these and other diverse traditions, I saw more clearly many more similarities even though the terminologies are different, even though some stated principles and objectives appear contradictory. They all are basically pointing in one direction: Sexuality is an essential part of our beingness.

Some label this general approach as *sacred sex* or *spiritual sex*, sometimes *Taoist sex*, but *tantra* seems to be emerging as the most popular nomenclature for many of us in the modern Western world who are seeking deeper meaning in both our sexual and spiritual dimensions. Some writers prefer *neo-Tantra*, since much of modern Western tantra is not traditional as written in the *Tantras*, an extensive set of scriptures in the East.

I have elected to use *tantra* with a lower case initial *t* to encompass any teachings and practices that are in alignment with the basic perspectives set forth in this Introduction. Included, for example, would be teachings from ancient peoples of the Americas and pre-Church-of-Rome religions in Europe. My apologies to anyone offended to find his or her tradition classified by a foreign concept. I feel life is served more by discovering the essential truths we have in common than by emphasizing differences in technique, language, cosmology, and tradition.

The Essential Tantra that follows is mainly my personal blend of themes and techniques with influences from these many approaches as well as my own discoveries. The eight meditation practices in the last section are from five nonincarnated beings, and thus from no tradition with which I am familiar.

I have made no attempt to teach traditional tantric ceremonies from third-century India. Our belief systems, technologies, and lifestyles are so different in the modern West. When a strictly vegetarian Brahman of almost two thousand years ago in India was confronted, for example, with a standard tantric ritual of eating various symbolic foods including meat, this novice had indeed run face-to-face into a poisonous plant in the middle of the path. For many of us today, the meat would be just another hamburger.

Since *The Essential Tantra* is a book and not a live interaction as in my seminars, I have not attempted to set any poisonous plants in these pages. To the contrary, "soft, sensual, cuddly" would characterize much of the text. The senses, obviously, are essential to every section. The possibility of sexual feelings and actions is always embraced. The choice not to be sexually active is always accepted.

Ceremony underlies many of the methods that follow. When we bring a sense of ceremony to our sensual-sexual expression, we are more apt to come into the present moment, allowing all the energies to become integrated into a wholeness.

Honoring our partner is the cornerstone of this book. Without choice and consensus, we have only manipulation; we have no real celebration. As our graspings and avoidings around our sexuality diminish, our soul can more easily commune with another. Truly allowing another to be exactly who and what she or he is at that moment, without attempting to change the other, is the ultimate honoring.

While the illustrations and language here often imply male-female twosomes, most of the techniques are applicable or easily adaptable to multiple-people situations and same-sex partners. In our sex life and life in general, homophobia and heterophobia are among the most limiting attachments we can have. Consuming that poisonous plant can be one of our most liberating actions to embrace the sexual and the spiritual.

Each moment, each action, each partner is a choice. We can make the choice consciously and dance in the center of the sacred circle. Or not.

When we embrace all of our sexuality,
we honor our spirituality.

When we embrace all of our spirituality,
we honor our sexuality.

When we embrace both, we celebrate God.

Tantric Massage

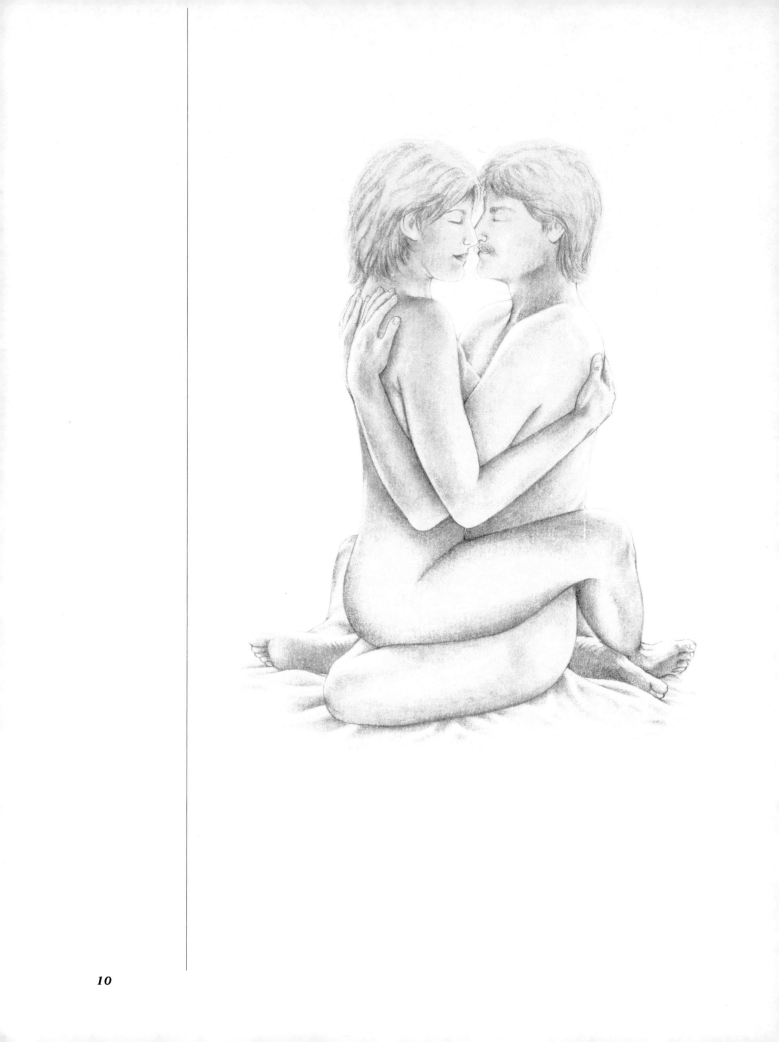

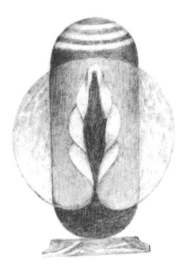

INVITATION

This is a language
without words

This is a time
outside of time

This is a song
that sings
a celebration

This is the meditation of massage

INTRODUCTION

Massage
    is a dance of energy

Massage
    is a dance of love

This is a love book especially for lovers
    Your boyfriend, your girlfriend
    your wife
    your husband
    your significant other, your lover, your mate
        the label is not important
    the feeling is

You may be friends
    exploring becoming lovers

You may be lovers
    exploring becoming friends

What is most important
        is that
what you do
    is
consensual

Massage simply stated
            simply is
        patterned touch
We might say
        a caress
        is unpatterned touch
Which you choose to give
        or to receive
        depends on the mood
Be open to either
        Both heal
        Both nurture
        Both excite

During the massage
        either or both of you
            might feel erotic
        You might fall asleep
        You might burst out in laughter
            or in tears

You might or might not
        have sex before
            during
            or after
        However, should sex or orgasm become
            the goal,
        you might miss
        many other pleasures

Allow each moment
            each feeling
        to unfold
        itself
This is the meditation

Massage
        is an art
                when you
        express yourself
                with sensitivity
                with awareness

Let your touch
discover
        without demands
        without expectations

At first
        the techniques
        will be
        techniques,
                like learning
                to ride a bicycle
After a while
        the awkward will become
        familiar

Your touch
        will come
        to nourish
the body
the mind
        and
the spirit

You will also find
        your beloved's body
                — in stillness —
        pleasuring your hands
Let your fingertips
        taste
                the curve
                the rough, the smooth
                the firm
                the soft

Let yourself feel

WHAT YOU NEED

A willing recipient

A quiet place

A warm place
      or if it is tropical,
      gentle breezes

Oil, perhaps a lotion
      — on membranous tissue,
           a water-based lubricant
           may be healthier

A towel

A padded table
      a bed or padded floor
      or a large towel
          on the beach

Gentle music, if you wish

Perhaps
      feathers
      a silk scarf

MEDITATIVE MASSAGE
GUIDELINES

Three basic ones:

First and foremost
    be present
Letting go of expectations
    of the future
        and
    comparisons with the past,
Be
    Here
Be
    Now

Secondly
    maintain full-hand contact
        whenever possible
    Allow your palms
        fingers
        and thumbs
    to outline the contours

Thirdly
    maintain a continuous flow
Movements blend together,
    each one
    enhancing the preceding one
    and preparing the next

More important
> than the techniques
> > is
> your own personal expression

More important than
> your own personal expression
> > is
> the recipient's wishes

More important than
> the recipient's wishes
> > is
> your never forcing yourself

Yet
> be open to discovering
> new horizons

It's a delicate dance

REMINDERS

If the sensation
      feels good to the recipient,
      you are doing it correctly,
         regardless
         of theory or written instructions

Vary
      the pressure
      the tempo
      the rhythm
Repeating a stroke in the exact same way each time
      becomes boring very quickly
      to both the recipient and the giver

If there are two of them,
      massage both

Glide on and off
      To begin a touch,
         rather than plopping on
      glide on with a slow descent
         in the direction
         that your hands will be moving
      In coming off
         continue the movement in a gradual ascent

Generally, minimize landings and takeoffs

When in doubt
      lighter pressure might be better
The recipient's preference, however,
      is the best guide
      Ask occasionally, if you are uncertain

Minimize the talking
An important exception:
    when the recipient needs
    to communicate deep feelings

Become centered
    Tuning into and slowing your breath
        you can quieten yourself

Being centered
    you will experience more deeply
    your own pleasure

The following strokes assume
    the massage is on a table
Except for some of the long strokes
    most of the instructions can be adapted
    to floor or bed massages

Follow the presented sequence
    or create a sequence
    more suitable for your situation

Massage the whole body
    or only one section

HEALTH

Discussing health concerns
>is essential
>in establishing trust
>in a relationship,
>>whether it be for an evening
>>or a lifetime

If a partner has a cold or flu,
>the other partner can choose
>to be close
>or not

If there is an infectious condition on the skin,
>forgo contact with that area
>Perhaps keep it clothed

If there is a concern
>about viral conditions
>communicable through bodily fluids,
>>share your feelings with your partner
>Read this book's appendix,
>>*Eroticizing Safer-Sex*
>Consult agencies promoting healthy sex
>>and read literature
>>which can assist you in choosing for yourself
>>what is best
>>in your sensual and sexual expressions

Ask if there are any tender places
Be especially gentle there
>or exclude
If an injury is severe
>or if there are circulation problems,
>first consult a health professional

The debates continue
      regarding the relative healthiness
      of vegetable oil
            mineral oil
            and water-based lubricants
      for massage on or in the body
Many commercial preparations contain
      preservatives, artificial colors
            and other chemical additives
      Some people are allergic
            to added fragrances
You may have to experiment first

Regarding conception
      please make parenthood planned

Now you are ready
      to make the final preparations
      for your special gift

PREPARATIONS

Where?

Anywhere
>> as long as distractions
>> and interruptions
>>> are minimized

Inside or outside is fine
>> When outside,
>>> take precautions
>>> for insects and excessive sun
>> When inside,
>>> unplug the phone
>> Arrange for everyone else
>>> including children
>> not to interrupt

It is very important
>> to maintain a warm temperature
>> If necessary, use a portable heater
>>> or cover the areas of the body
>>> you are not massaging at the moment

When?

Explore the energies of
>> a full moon, a new moon
>> an equinox, a solstice

Celebrate a birthday
>>> an anniversary
>> Give a holiday-season present
>>> handmade

After intense work
>> during a stressful period

Sometimes you can be spontaneous
      but setting aside a specific day or evening
         is more likely
         to ensure it happening

To give massage to a pregnant partner,
      is a gift not forgotten
   In the later stages
      she may be unable to lie on her front or back
   Perhaps forego some strokes or positions
      but not the touch

With What?

Basically all you need is oil
        fragranced ones entice the mind
           but may sting the skin
           especially membranous tissue
Some prefer vegetable oils
        (unfragranced coconut oil is a good choice)
        others prefer mineral oils
           Visit your local lotions-and-potions store,
              try a health food store
On membranous tissues, such as the female genitals,
        some consider water-based lubricants
        to be healthier
           Purchase them at a pharmacy
           perhaps at a sensuous boutique
You can apply the oil or lubricant to your hands
        either from a plastic squeeze bottle
        a bottle with a push pump
        or a bowl

Massage tables are great for your back
        and sturdy tabletops
           padded with foam or blankets are fine
        Otherwise, a padded floor
          a bed
          or the ground covered with cloth
          is quite suitable

If you select a large bed
        have the recipient's head
           at a corner of the foot of the bed
           while his/her feet are pointing toward
           the opposite corner at the head of the bed
        This will give you better access
          to both the right and left sides

For the covering cloth
        select a sheet or material
        that is OK to be oiled
           Some fabrics are difficult to clean
          and the oily smell may not wash out

Gather a large towel or two

When lying on the front side
        the recipient may need a covered foam pad
                or a couple of rolled towels
        placed under the front of the ankles

When lying on the back
        if there is strain in the lower back
        place the same pad underneath the knees

If you anticipate using feathers
                or other tactile stimulators
        have them close at hand

Perhaps select some music
        without dominating rhythms
        without words — usually

Use candlelight or colored lights
        incense
        flowers
        interior design of the room
                or whatever creates a special ambience
        However
        you do not have to create a temple every time
Sometimes
        all that is necessary
                is
        to close the door

Everything ready?

Oil

> phone unplugged
> temperature warm enough
> watches, jewelry, clothing removed
> recipient's contact lenses taken out (if necessary)
> your fingernails smoothed
> your hands cleaned and warmed?

Ask if any strokes
> on any particular places
> would be particularly pleasing

Ask for other possible relevancies
> such as preferences for no oil in the hair
> or time limitations

Once your beloved
> > is ready to begin
> give the invitation
> > to take a few fuller breaths
> > > and
> > to close his/her eyes

Allowing
> > your hands
> > to move intuitively
> you can open doors
> > to inner peace
> > to pleasure
> > to joy
> both your beloved's
> > and
> yours

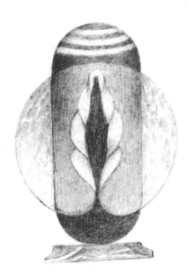

THE
MASSAGE
THE
MEDITATION

BEGINNING

Lover's Position: Lying front down with arms by side.
Your Position: Initially at your lover's left side.

1. Laying On Of Hands
1. A

1. Laying On Of Hands

A.
Center yourself.
Tune into your breathing.

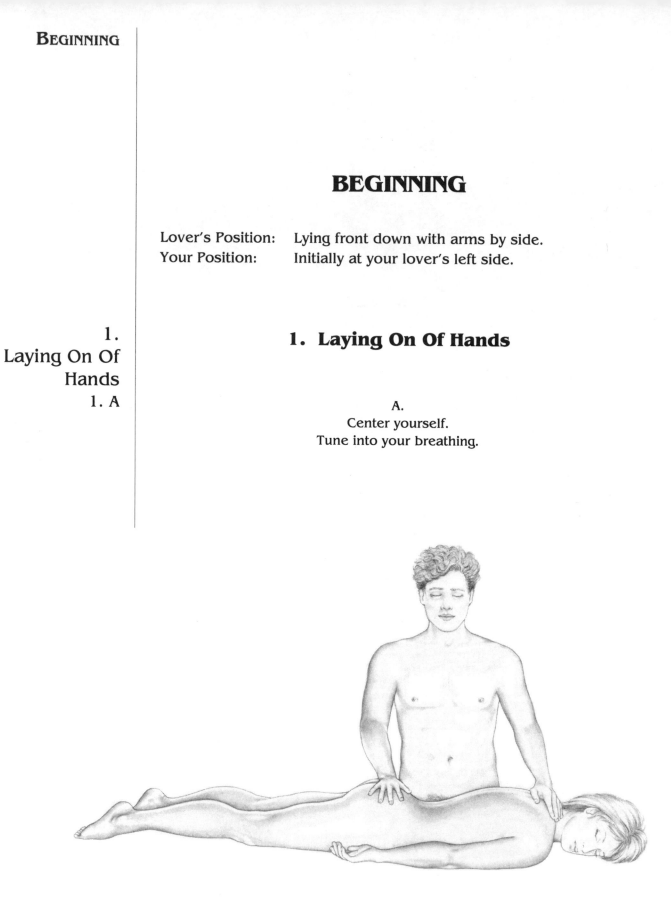

1. B

B.
Rest your left palm on the upper back,
your right palm on the sacrum.

Laying On Of Hands

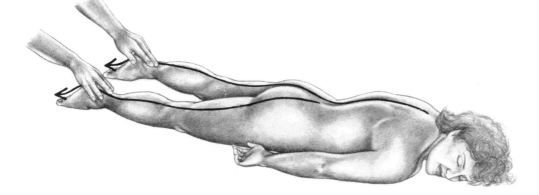

C.
Lightly pull your hands downward,
separating at the waist
and then flowing down off the tips of the toes.

If you have feathers
or other sensuous materials,
stroke your lover
— all over —
now
before you apply any oil.

1. C

2. Spreading Oil

A.
Warm oil in your hands.
(Be careful not to let drops fall on your partner.)

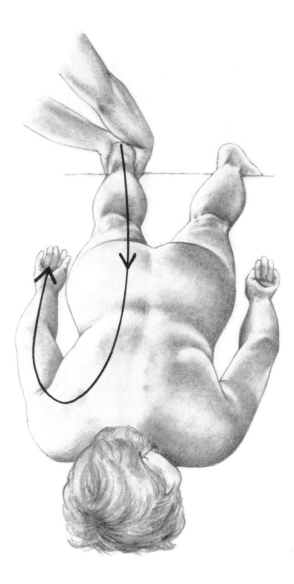

B.
Spread the oil by sliding your hands
up the back side:
starting at the feet, pull up the legs, the torso,
all the way off the fingertips.

~

Repeat the same sequence on the other side.
(It is easier if you first move to the other side.)

This is not the only oil application.
Generally, you add more oil
in the initial stroke of each section.

BACK

Your Position: Initially at your lover's head and facing his/her feet.

3. Connecting Stroke

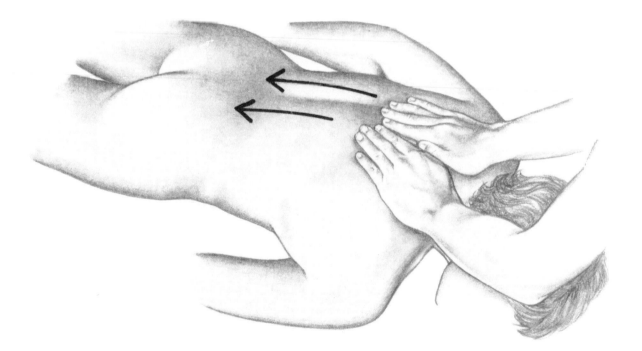

A.
Slide your parallel palms down the back
to the buttocks.

3. A

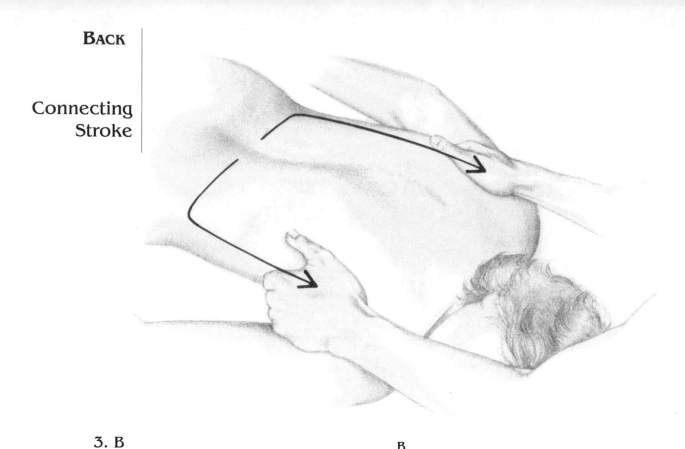

3. B

B.
Slide your palms outward to the sides of the waist
and then up the sides to the shoulders.

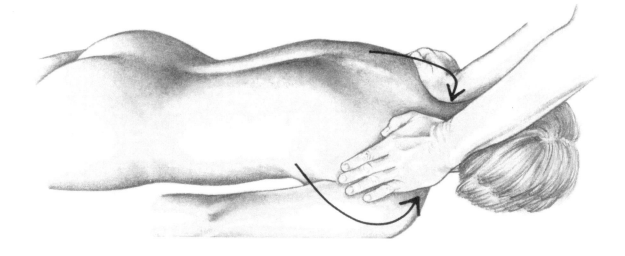

3. C

C.
On the shoulders, pivot your hands outward.

Connecting
Stroke

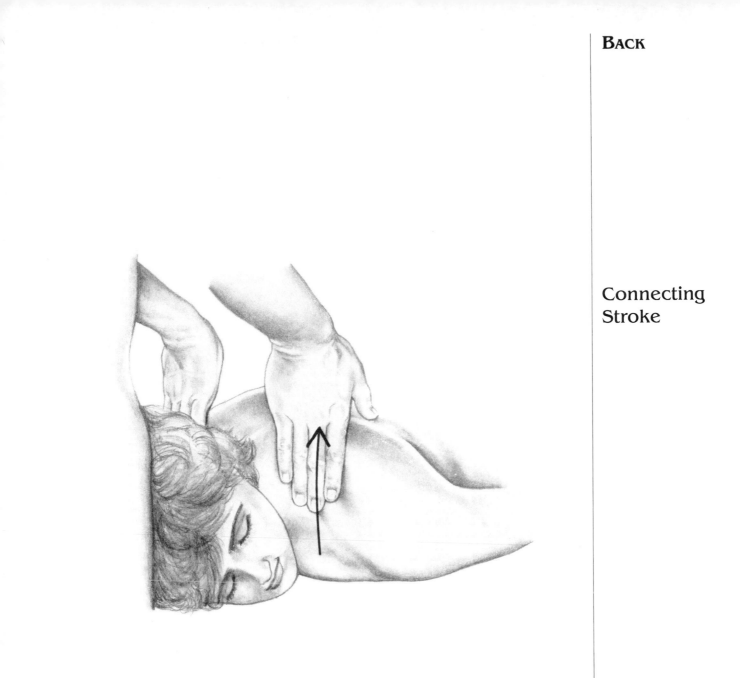

D.
Slide upwards across the shoulder muscles
(not the throat).

~

Repeat this whole stroke (A-D) several times.

3. D

4. Prayer Stroke

4.
Prayer Stroke

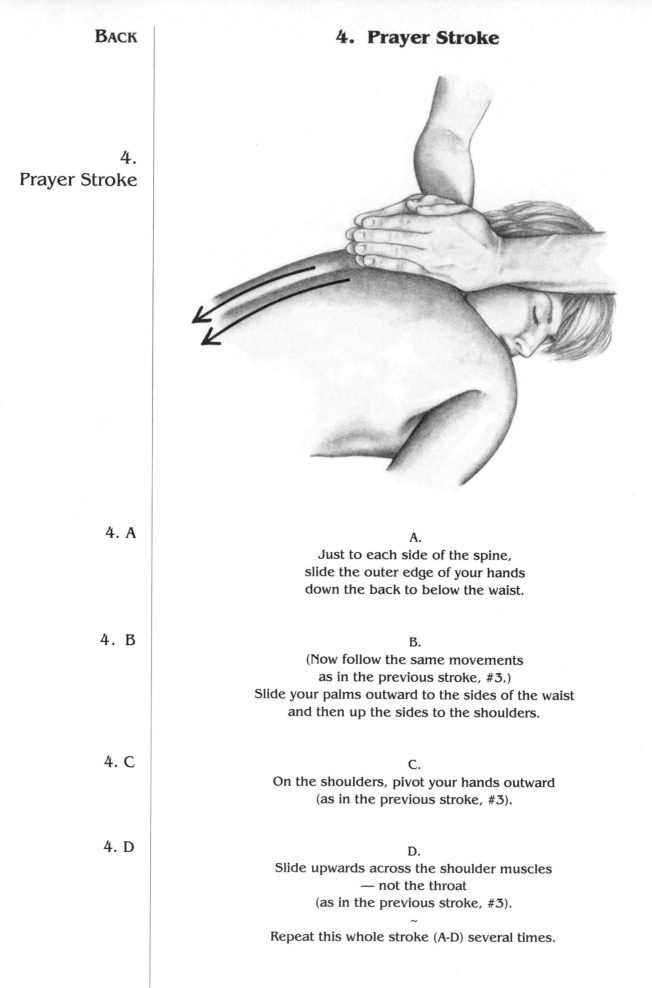

4. A

A.
Just to each side of the spine,
slide the outer edge of your hands
down the back to below the waist.

4. B

B.
(Now follow the same movements
as in the previous stroke, #3.)
Slide your palms outward to the sides of the waist
and then up the sides to the shoulders.

4. C

C.
On the shoulders, pivot your hands outward
(as in the previous stroke, #3).

4. D

D.
Slide upwards across the shoulder muscles
— not the throat
(as in the previous stroke, #3).
~
Repeat this whole stroke (A-D) several times.

5. Shoulder Strokes

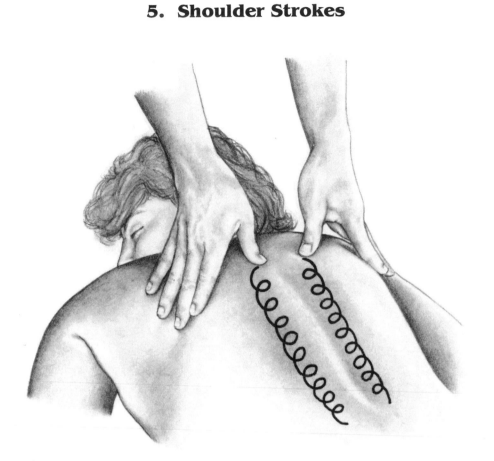

A.
Just to each side of the spine,
make circles with the flat parts of your thumbs.
Here the thumbs mirror each other:
down together,
outward from spine together,
etc.

Focus the pressure
in the direction toward his/her feet.
Let your fingers remain in contact with your partner.

This series of circles gradually comes UP the back.

Shoulder Strokes

5. B

B.
On the right shoulder
between the spine and scapula,
make circles with your thumbs
— this time alternating your hands
one after the other.

Focus on the area near the neck.

Shoulder
Strokes

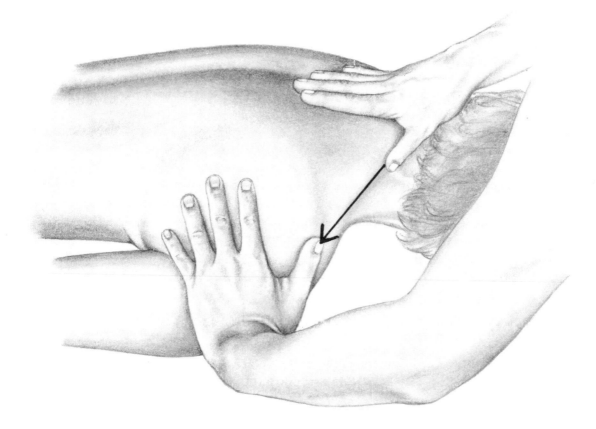

C.
On the groove
between the right scapula and clavicle,
slide your thumbs outward toward the shoulder tip
— alternating one hand after the other.

5. C

D.
Now apply Parts B and C on the left shoulder.

5. D

6.
Fingers' Pull

6. Fingers' Pull

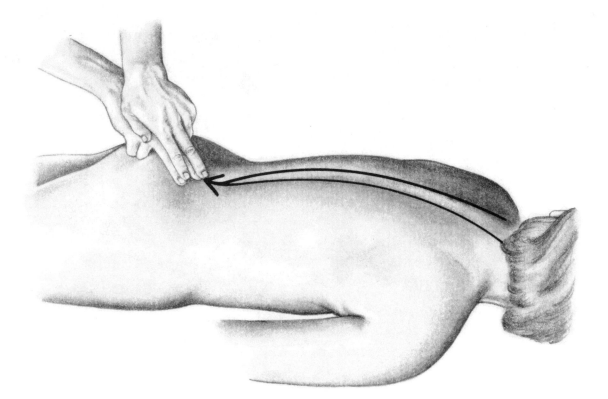

With a finger pad
on each side of the spine at the neck,
pull downward toward the buttocks.
Use a firm pressure.
(You can have even more pressure
by putting the fingers of your other hand
on top of the first.)

~

Repeat this whole stroke several times.

7. Side Pulling

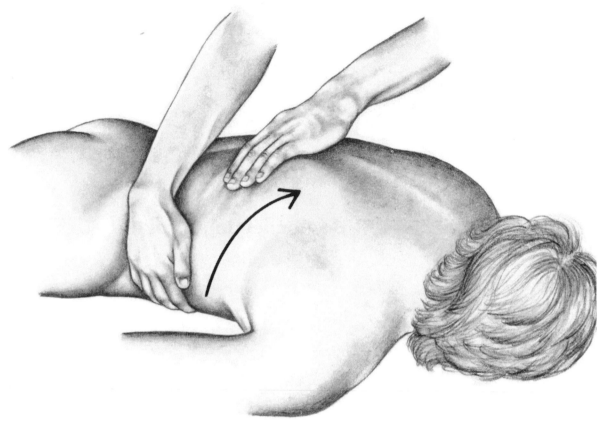

A.
Alternating your hands on one side,
slide them in a pulling manner
across the side of the torso
toward the spine.

(This series includes the area from the hips
to near the underarms.)

B.
Move to the other side,
and apply the pulling movements
to the opposite side.

BACK OF LEGS

Instructions: Written as applied to the right leg.
Your Position: Initially, to the right of the right foot.

**8.
Connecting
Stroke**

8. Connecting Stroke

A.
With your right hand in front,
slide your hands up the back of the leg.

(For both hands, the little-finger-side leads;
the thumbs are beside their index fingers.)

8. A

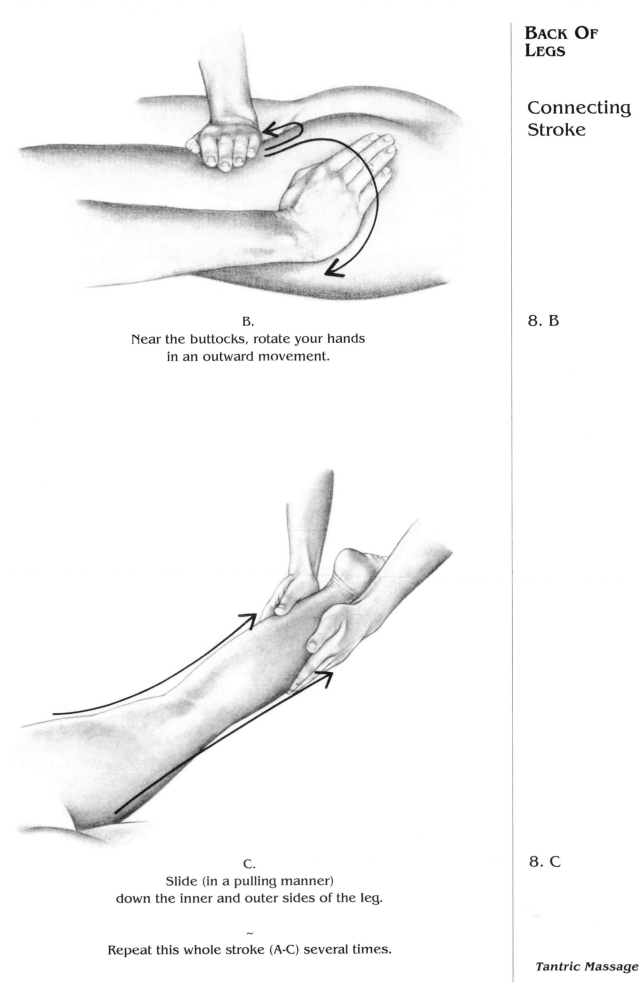

B.
Near the buttocks, rotate your hands
in an outward movement.

8. B

C.
Slide (in a pulling manner)
down the inner and outer sides of the leg.

~
Repeat this whole stroke (A-C) several times.

8. C

9. Kneading

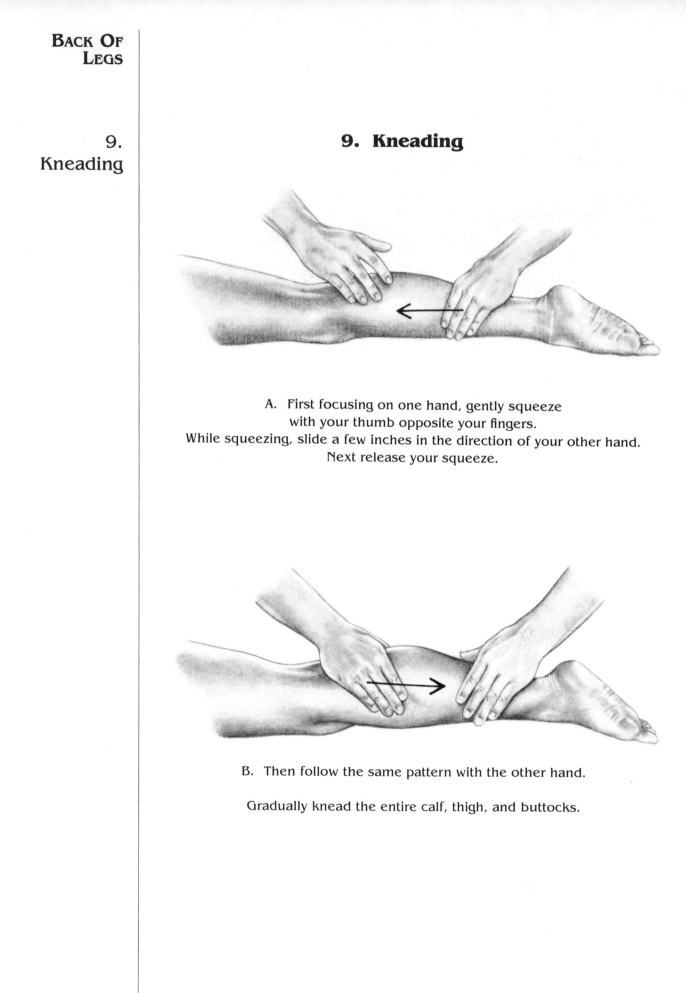

A. First focusing on one hand, gently squeeze
with your thumb opposite your fingers.
While squeezing, slide a few inches in the direction of your other hand.
Next release your squeeze.

B. Then follow the same pattern with the other hand.

Gradually knead the entire calf, thigh, and buttocks.

10. Thumb Slide

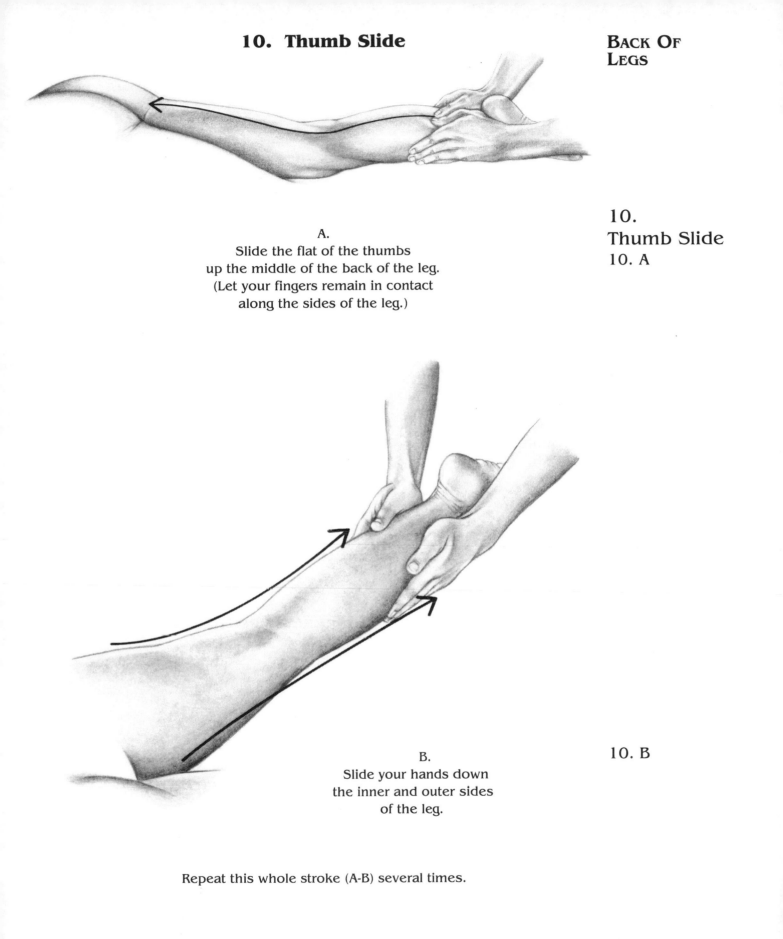

A.
Slide the flat of the thumbs
up the middle of the back of the leg.
(Let your fingers remain in contact
along the sides of the leg.)

B.
Slide your hands down
the inner and outer sides
of the leg.

Repeat this whole stroke (A-B) several times.

11. V Stroke

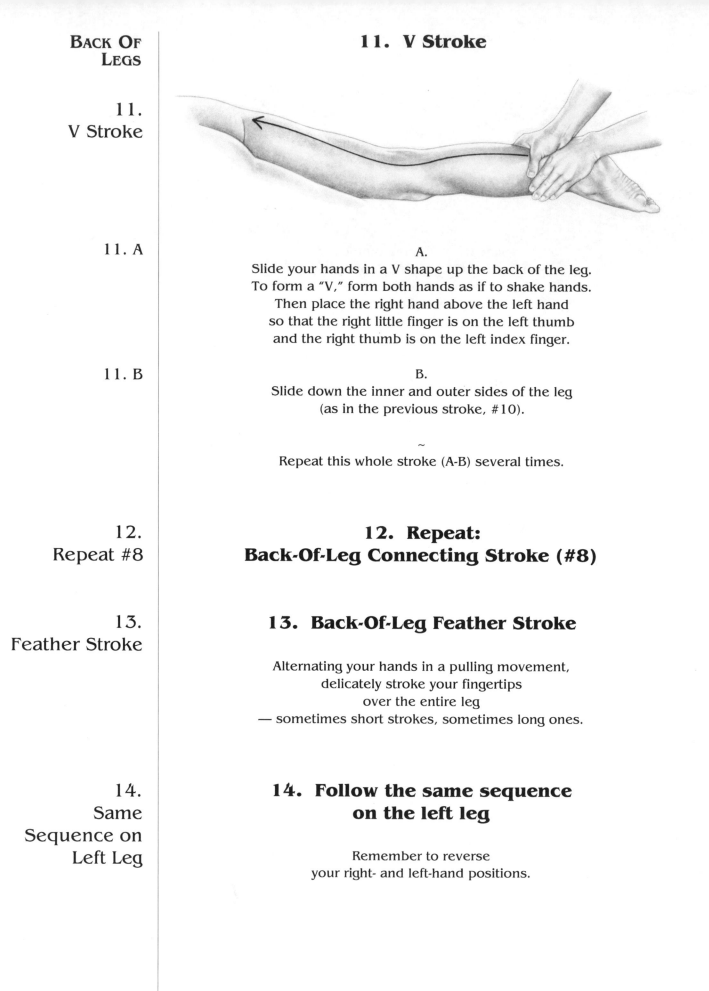

A.
Slide your hands in a V shape up the back of the leg.
To form a "V," form both hands as if to shake hands.
Then place the right hand above the left hand
so that the right little finger is on the left thumb
and the right thumb is on the left index finger.

B.
Slide down the inner and outer sides of the leg
(as in the previous stroke, #10).

~

Repeat this whole stroke (A-B) several times.

12. Repeat:
Back-Of-Leg Connecting Stroke (#8)

13. Back-Of-Leg Feather Stroke

Alternating your hands in a pulling movement,
delicately stroke your fingertips
over the entire leg
— sometimes short strokes, sometimes long ones.

14. Follow the same sequence
on the left leg

Remember to reverse
your right- and left-hand positions.

BACK SIDE CONCLUSION

15. Back Hug

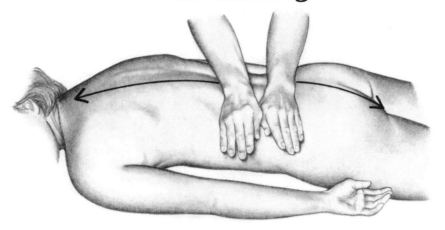

A.
(This may be a difficult stroke
unless you are using a massage table.)

Using the soft, inner side of your forearms,
begin at your lover's lower back
and slide them to below the buttocks
and to the upper back.

Then slide your forearms back together.
~
Repeat this whole movement several times.

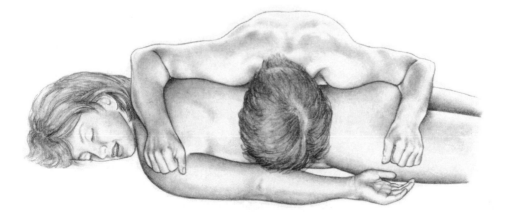

B.
After a few repetitions of Part A,
rest your chest on the back.

Be very careful
not to put pressure on the neck and throat area.

16. Concluding Stroke

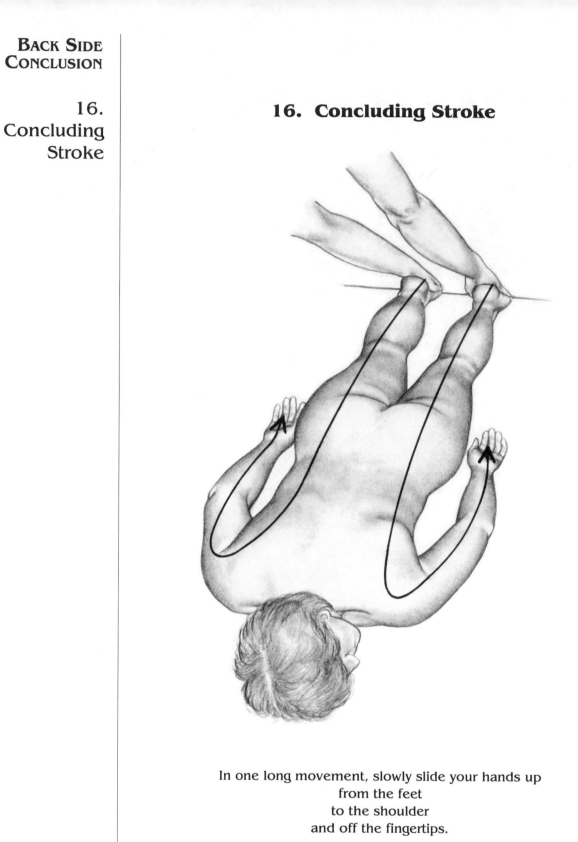

In one long movement, slowly slide your hands up
from the feet
to the shoulder
and off the fingertips.

If you wish, then gently feather stroke
with your fingertips
the entire back side.

~

After a while, with a gentle voice,
invite your lover to turn over when ready.

ARMS

Instructions: Written as applied to the right arm.
Lover's Position: Lying on back with arms by side.
Your Position: Initially at the right waist, facing the head.

17. Connecting Stroke

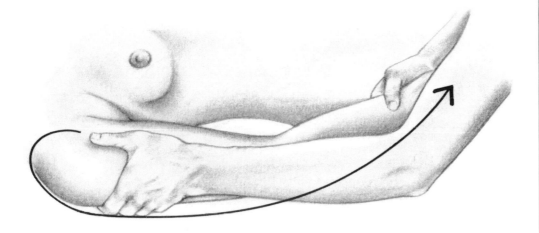

A.
First, gently hold the right wrist in your right hand.
Then with the little finger side leading,
slide your left hand up
the outside of the right arm.

B.
Pivot on the shoulder tip
and slide down
on the back side of the arm.

**Connecting
Stroke**

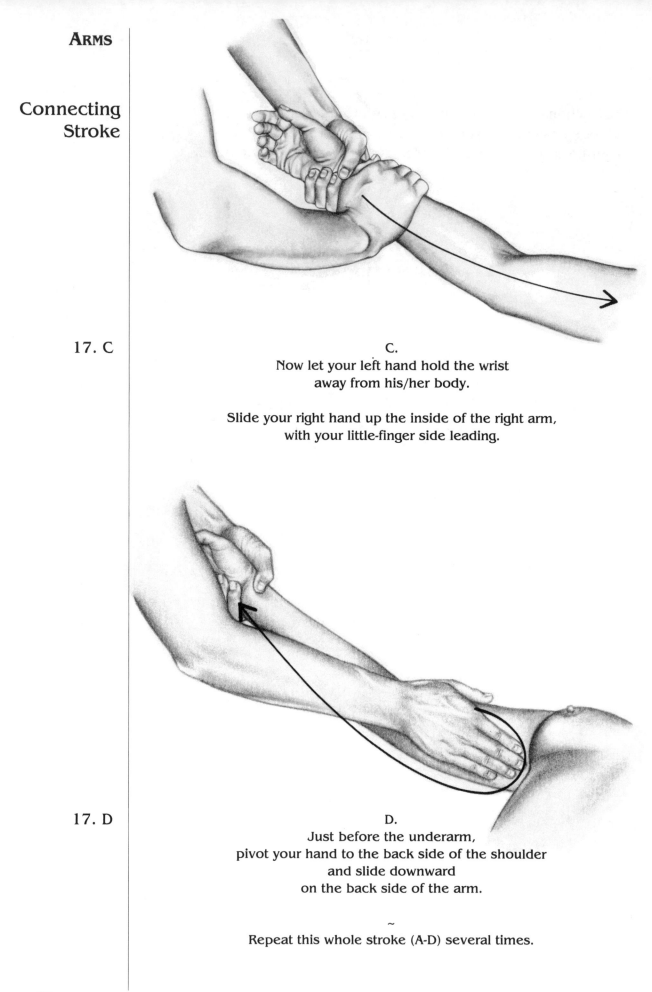

17. C

C.
Now let your left hand hold the wrist
away from his/her body.

Slide your right hand up the inside of the right arm,
with your little-finger side leading.

17. D

D.
Just before the underarm,
pivot your hand to the back side of the shoulder
and slide downward
on the back side of the arm.

~

Repeat this whole stroke (A-D) several times.

18. Upper Arm Stroke

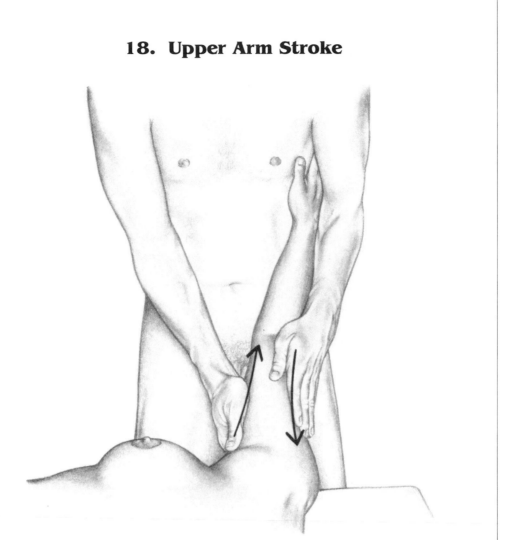

A.
Hold the right hand on your left rib cage.

Slide your left hand upward
on the outside of his/her upper arm

while your right hand slides downward
on the back side.

18. A

Upper Arm Stroke

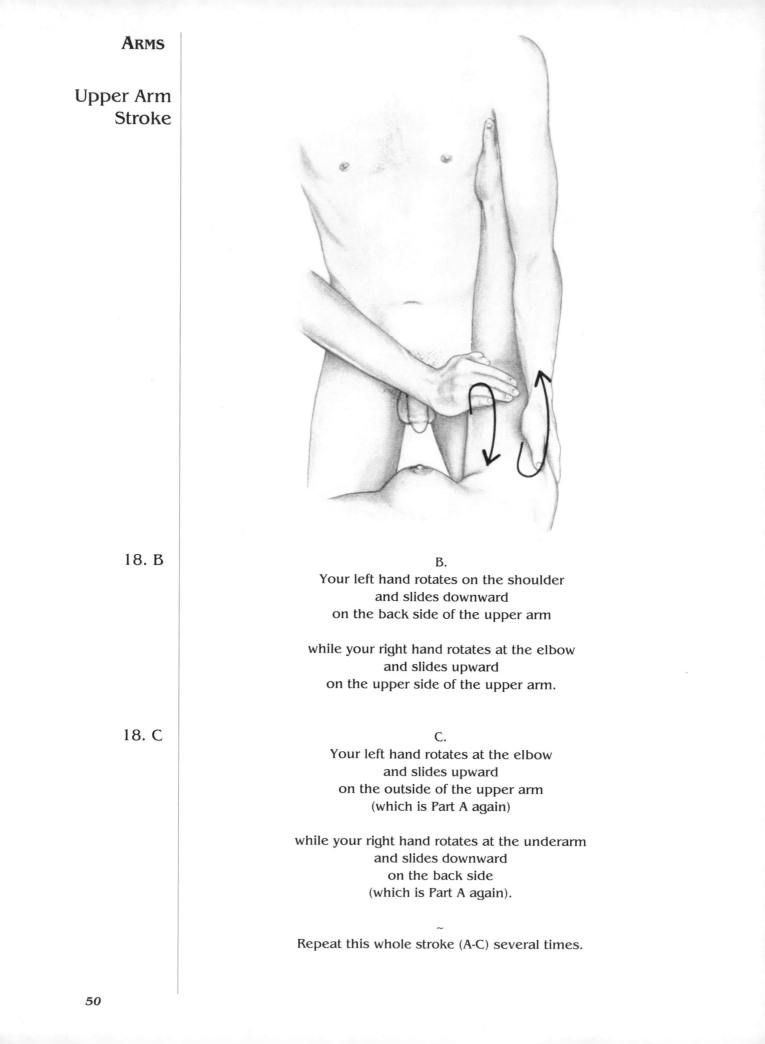

18. B

B.
Your left hand rotates on the shoulder
and slides downward
on the back side of the upper arm

while your right hand rotates at the elbow
and slides upward
on the upper side of the upper arm.

18. C

C.
Your left hand rotates at the elbow
and slides upward
on the outside of the upper arm
(which is Part A again)

while your right hand rotates at the underarm
and slides downward
on the back side
(which is Part A again).

~

Repeat this whole stroke (A-C) several times.

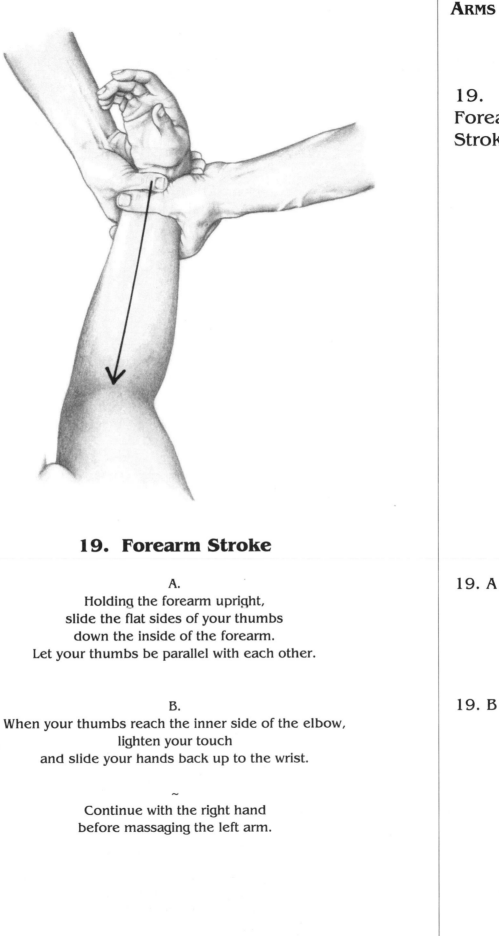

19. Forearm Stroke

A.
Holding the forearm upright,
slide the flat sides of your thumbs
down the inside of the forearm.
Let your thumbs be parallel with each other.

B.
When your thumbs reach the inner side of the elbow,
lighten your touch
and slide your hands back up to the wrist.

~
Continue with the right hand
before massaging the left arm.

HANDS

Instructions: Written as applied to the right hand.

20. Hand Curl

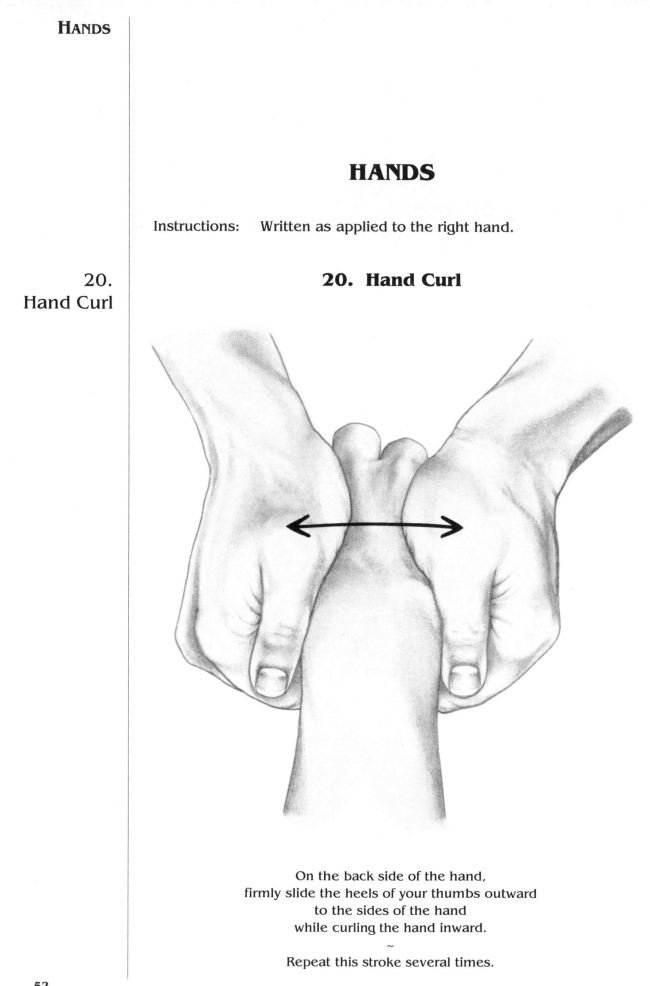

On the back side of the hand,
firmly slide the heels of your thumbs outward
to the sides of the hand
while curling the hand inward.

~

Repeat this stroke several times.

21. Palm Massage

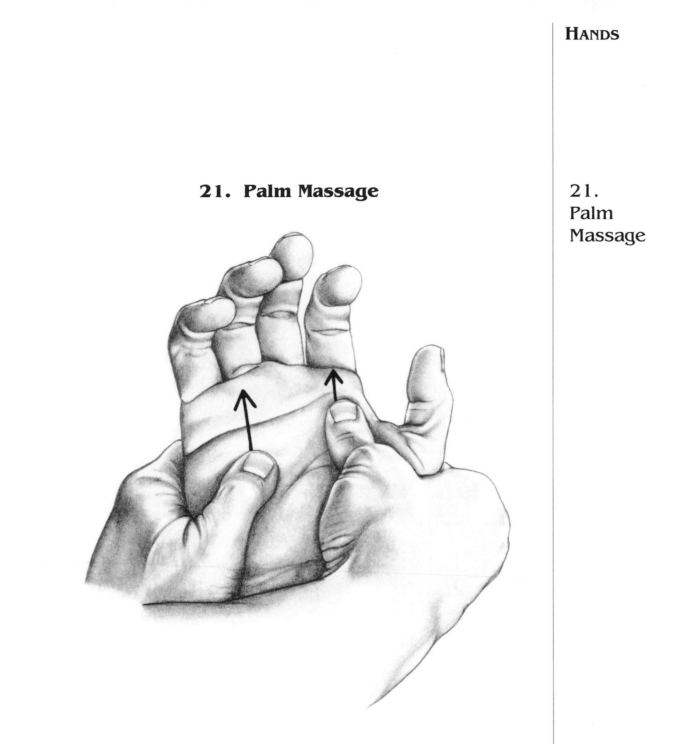

Alternating your thumbs,
firmly push your thumb pads upward on the palm.
Repeat the movements many times,
covering the palm entirely.

22.
Web Stroke

22. Web Stroke

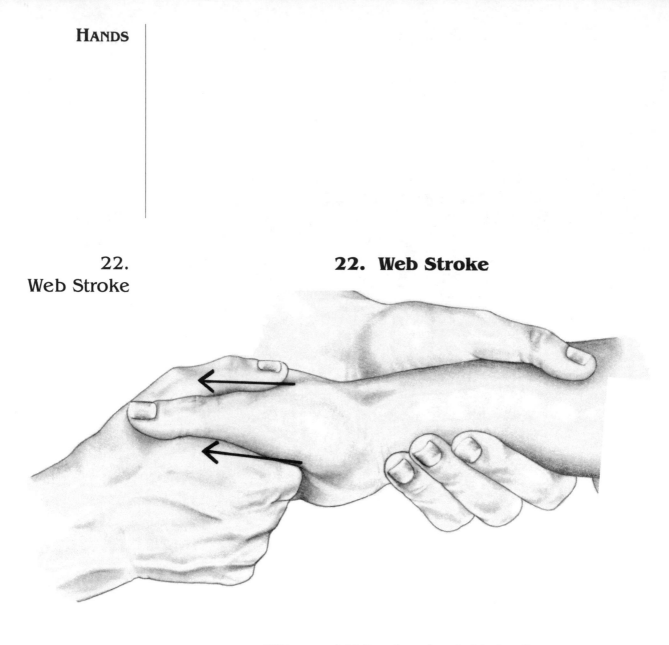

With your right thumb and curled index finger
between the right thumb and first finger,
slide outward firmly.

~

Repeat this stroke several times.

23. Finger Stroke

A.
Starting at the tip of the finger,
slide very lightly down the sides of the finger
with your thumb and finger
— very, very lightly.

B.
Grasping the finger firmly at its base,
slide up and off the finger.

~

Repeat Part A and Part B once on the thumb
and once on each finger.

24. Palm Reading

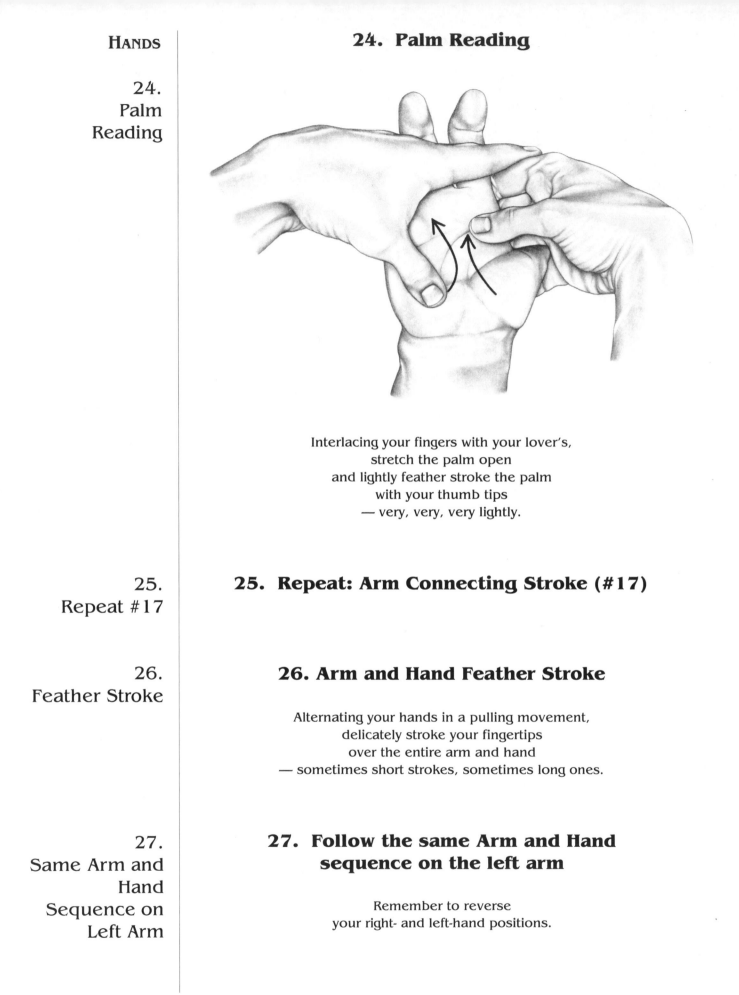

Interlacing your fingers with your lover's,
stretch the palm open
and lightly feather stroke the palm
with your thumb tips
— very, very, very lightly.

25. Repeat: Arm Connecting Stroke (#17)

26. Arm and Hand Feather Stroke

Alternating your hands in a pulling movement,
delicately stroke your fingertips
over the entire arm and hand
— sometimes short strokes, sometimes long ones.

27. Follow the same Arm and Hand sequence on the left arm

Remember to reverse
your right- and left-hand positions.

FRONT OF LEGS

Instructions: Written as applied to the right leg.

28. Connecting Stroke

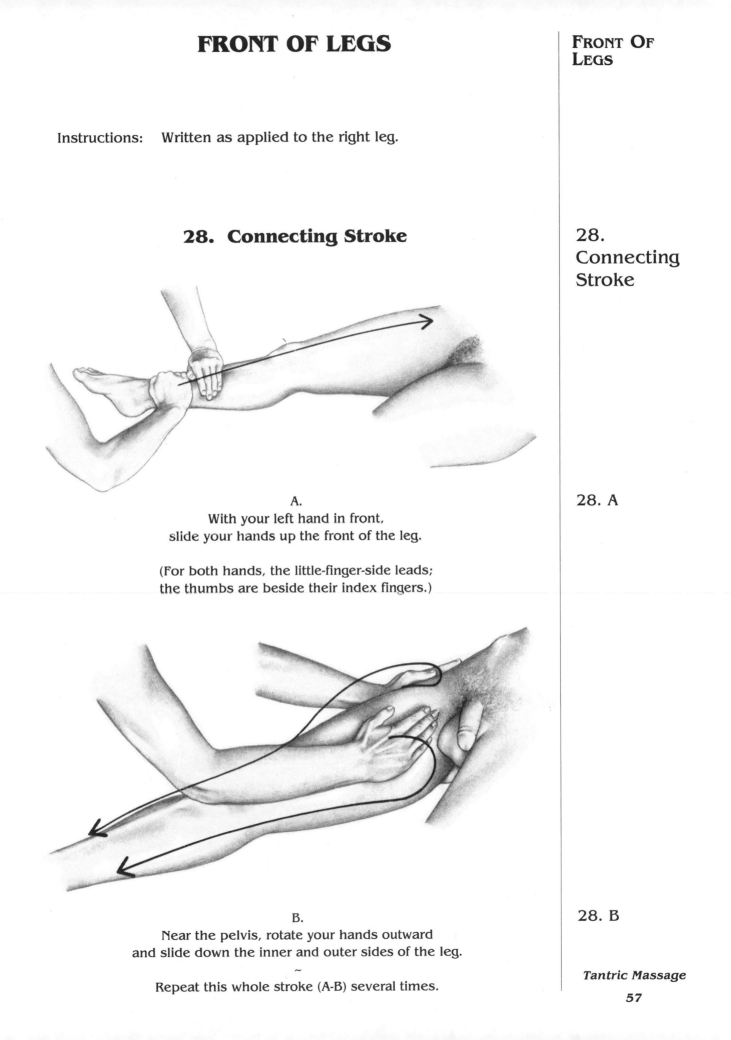

A.
With your left hand in front,
slide your hands up the front of the leg.

(For both hands, the little-finger-side leads;
the thumbs are beside their index fingers.)

B.
Near the pelvis, rotate your hands outward
and slide down the inner and outer sides of the leg.

~

Repeat this whole stroke (A-B) several times.

29.
Mini-
Connecting
Stroke

29. Mini-Connecting Stroke

On the thigh,
make a series of connecting strokes
similar to the previous stroke (#28)
but shorter and only on the thigh.

Each succeeding stroke starts
a little farther up the thigh
and ends a little farther up.
~
Repeat this whole series several times.

30. Thigh Kneading

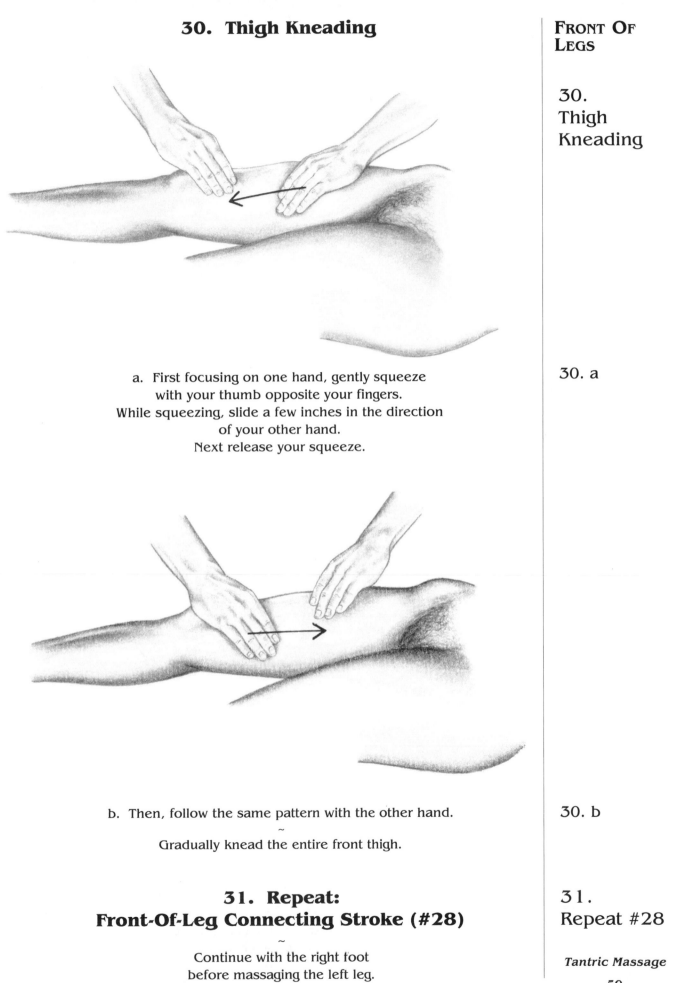

a. First focusing on one hand, gently squeeze
with your thumb opposite your fingers.
While squeezing, slide a few inches in the direction
of your other hand.
Next release your squeeze.

b. Then, follow the same pattern with the other hand.

~

Gradually knead the entire front thigh.

31. Repeat:
Front-Of-Leg Connecting Stroke (#28)

~

Continue with the right foot
before massaging the left leg.

FEET

32. Ankle Circling

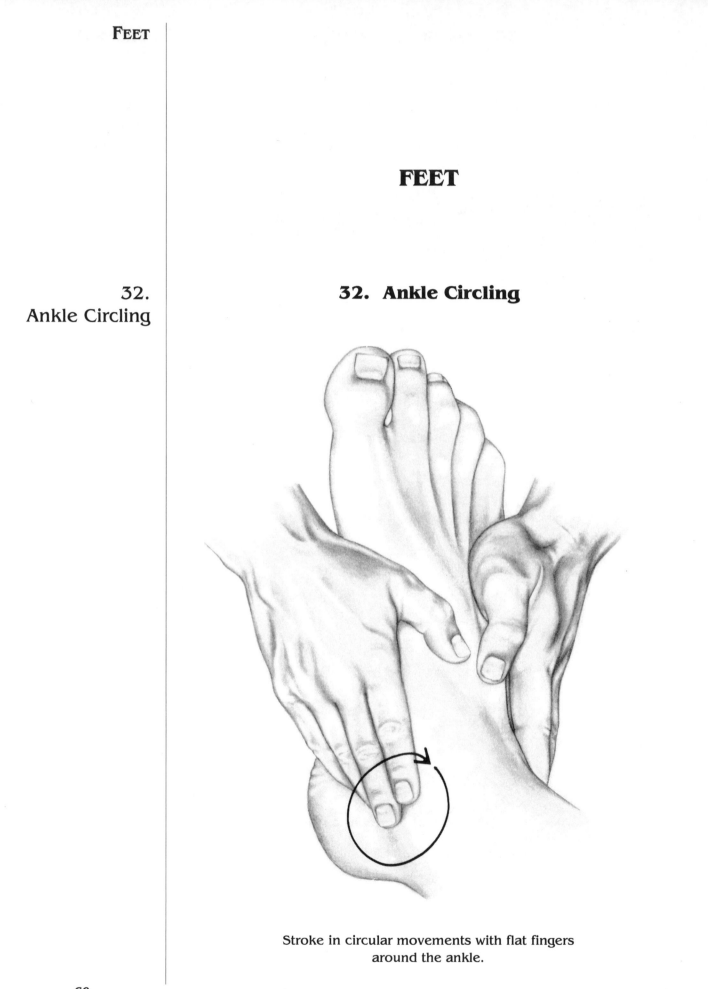

Stroke in circular movements with flat fingers
around the ankle.

33. Connecting Stroke

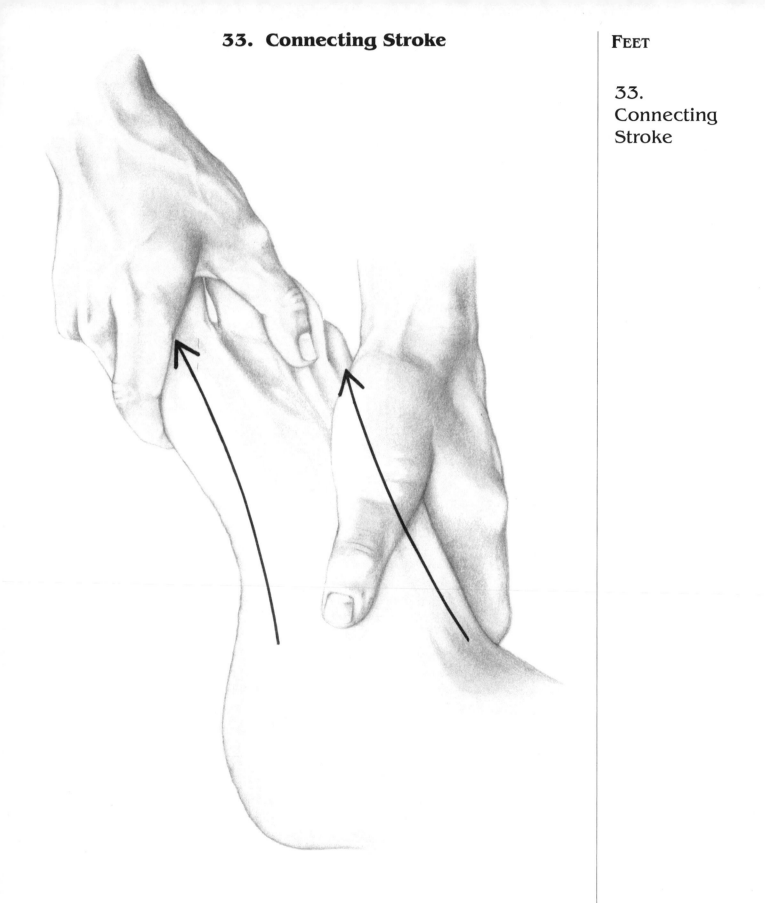

Alternating your hands,
squeeze the foot
and slide off the end.

~

Repeat this stroke several times.

34. Arc de Triomphe

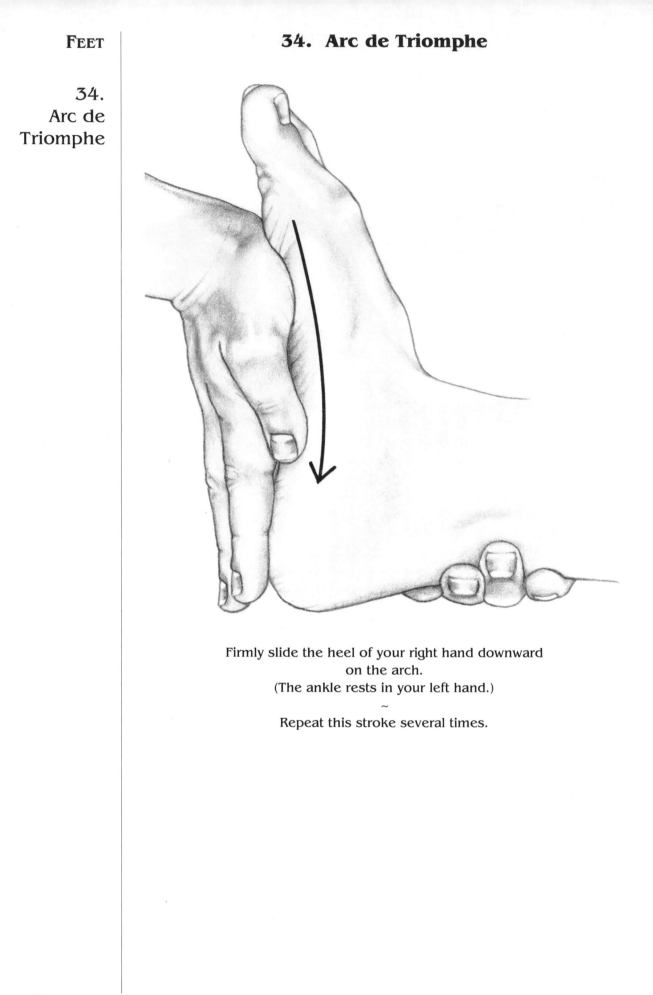

Firmly slide the heel of your right hand downward
on the arch.
(The ankle rests in your left hand.)

~

Repeat this stroke several times.

35. Finger Circles

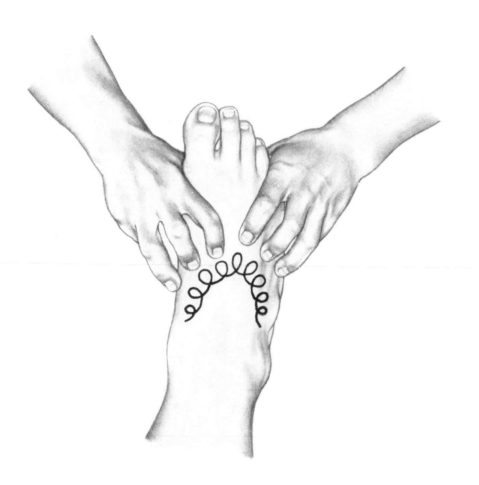

On the top of the foot,
make small circles with your finger pads.

(Slide your fingers over the skin
and/or, with a little more pressure,
slide your lover's skin over the muscles,
tendons, and bones beneath.)

~

Repeat these circles over the entire top of the foot.

36.
Between-The-
Toes Stroke

36. Between-The-Toes Stroke

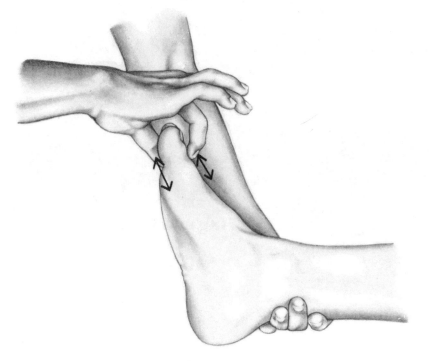

With your right-hand index finger
on top on the right foot
and your right-hand thumb on the bottom,
squeeze and slide up and down several times
between each of the toes.

37.
Slithering

37. Slithering

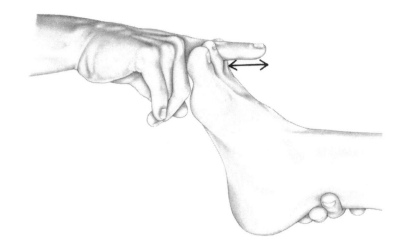

Very slowly and gently "screw" any right finger in and out
between each set of toes.

38. Repeat:
Front-Of-Leg Connecting Stroke (#28)

39. Leg and Foot Feather Stroke

Alternating your hands in a pulling movement,
delicately stroke your fingertips
over the entire leg and foot
— sometimes short strokes, sometimes long ones.

40. Follow the same Front-Of-Legs and Feet sequence on the left side

~
Remember to reverse
your right- and left-hand positions.

38.
Repeat #28

39.
Feather Stroke

40.
Same Front-Of-Legs and Feet Sequence on Left Side

FRONT TORSO

Your Position: Initially at your lover's right side.

41. Moon Stroke

41.
Moon Stroke:
practice

First, practice your right- and left-hand movements separately:

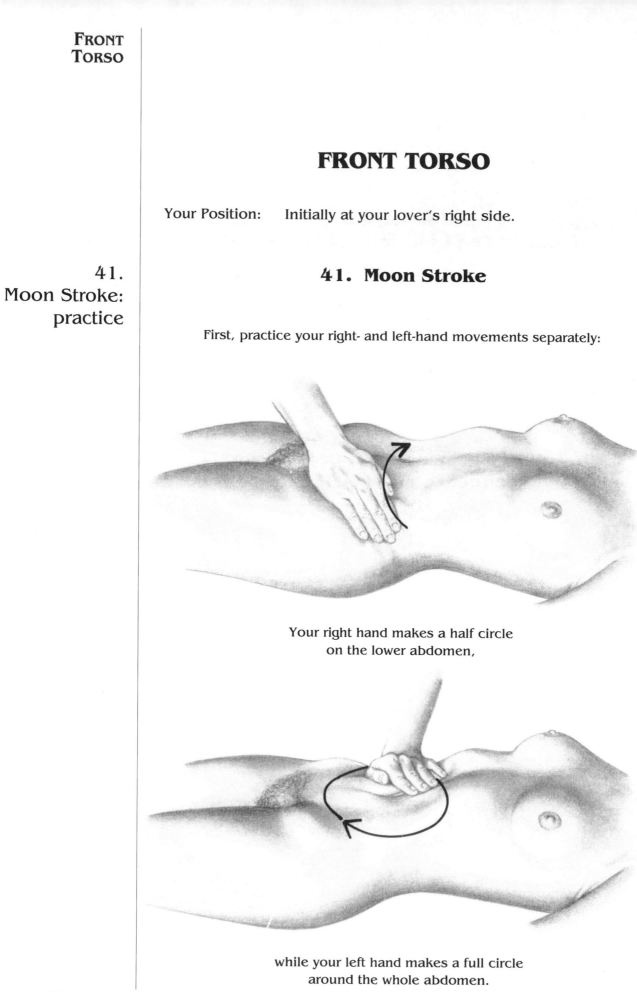

Your right hand makes a half circle
on the lower abdomen,

while your left hand makes a full circle
around the whole abdomen.

This is the complete version:

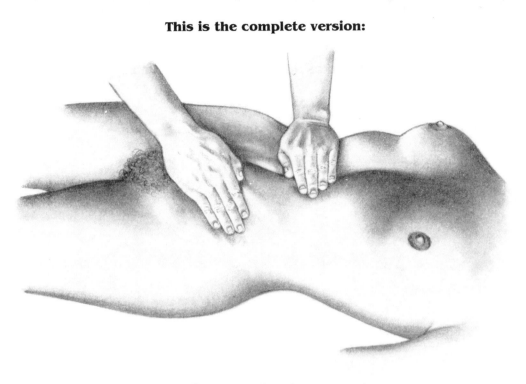

Front
Torso

41.
Moon Stroke:
complete
version

Coordinate your hand movements:
when your right hand is stroking in a half circle,
your left hand is directly opposite on the circle.

When not using your right hand,
simply lift it out of the way
of your left hand's full-circle pattern.

~

Repeat this whole stroke several times.

42. Center Slide

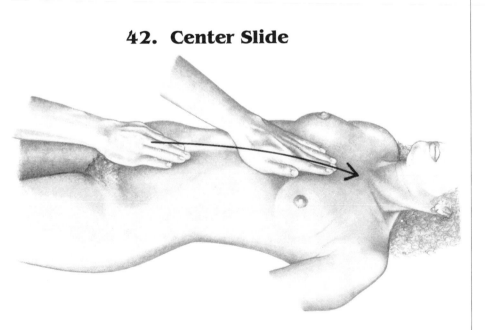

Alternating your hands,
firmly and slowly slide them up the midline
from the lower abdomen to the upper chest.

43. Breast Kneading

Instructions: Written as applied to the right breast.

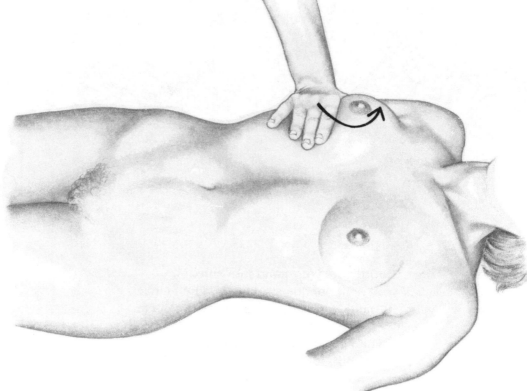

43. A

A.
Starting at the lower, outer side of the breast area,
slide your right hand up over the breast
so that your thumb and index finger
encircle the nipple.

Using the nipple as the axis,
continue the stroke
by rotating your hand counterclockwise
around the nipple
as you slide up and off the breast.

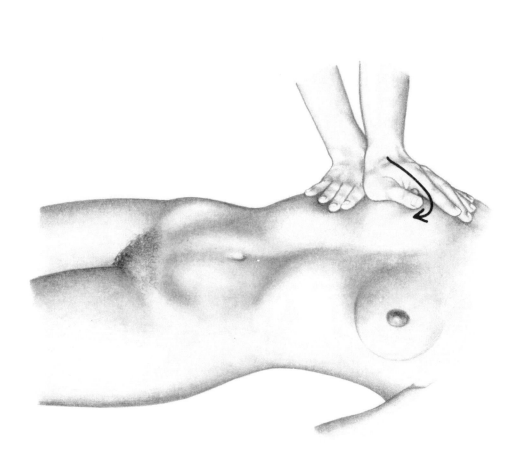

43. B

B.
Slide your left hand
from the same lower, outer side of the breast area
up over the breast
so that your thumb and index finger
encircle the nipple.

Using the nipple as the axis,
continue the stroke
by rotating your left hand clockwise
around the nipple
as you slide up and off the breast.

~

Repeat this series (A-B) several times
with one hand following the other.

~

Continue with the following stroke (#44)
on the right breast
before massaging the left breast.

Note:
On a woman's breast, apply a lighter pressure.

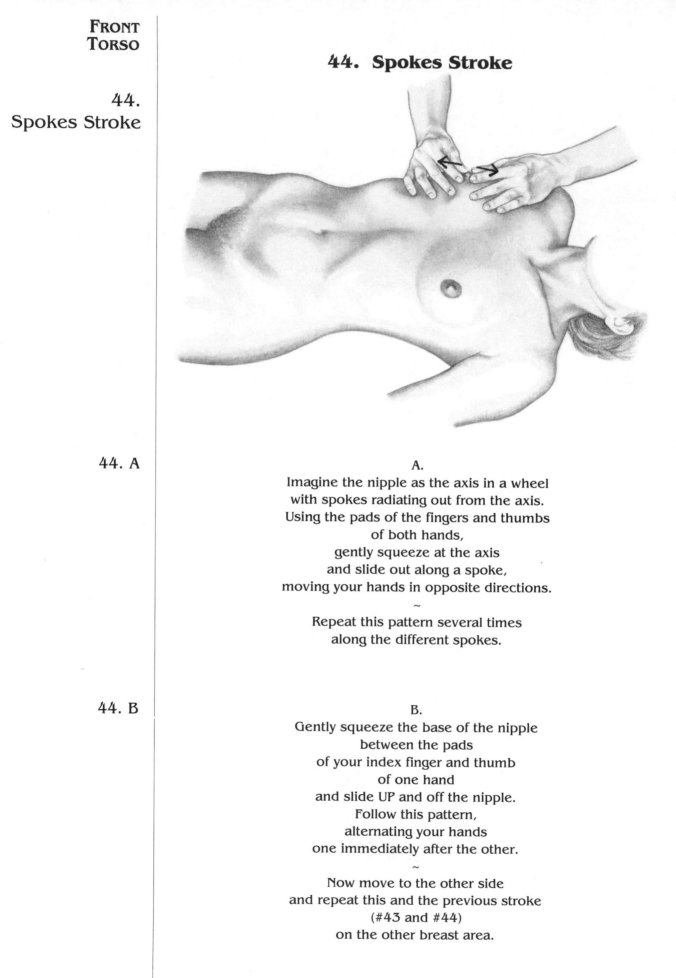

44. Spokes Stroke

44. A

A.
Imagine the nipple as the axis in a wheel
with spokes radiating out from the axis.
Using the pads of the fingers and thumbs
of both hands,
gently squeeze at the axis
and slide out along a spoke,
moving your hands in opposite directions.
~

Repeat this pattern several times
along the different spokes.

44. B

B.
Gently squeeze the base of the nipple
between the pads
of your index finger and thumb
of one hand
and slide UP and off the nipple.
Follow this pattern,
alternating your hands
one immediately after the other.
~

Now move to the other side
and repeat this and the previous stroke
(#43 and #44)
on the other breast area.

45. Side Pulling

A.
Alternating your hands,
slide them in a pulling manner
across the side of the torso
toward the front midline.

~

(This series includes the area
from the hips to near the underarms.
Be gentle on the mammary area.)

45. A

B.
Move to the other side,
and apply the pulling movements
to the opposite side.

45. B

46. Torso Feather Stroke

Alternating your hands in a pulling movement,
delicately stroke your fingertips
over the entire torso.
Include the genital and thigh areas as well.

46.
Torso Feather
Stroke

GENITALS: MALE

Lover's Position: Lying on back.
Your Position: To your lover's right side.
Note: If you wish to follow safer-sex practices, please
                     consult the appendix.

47. Anointing With Oil

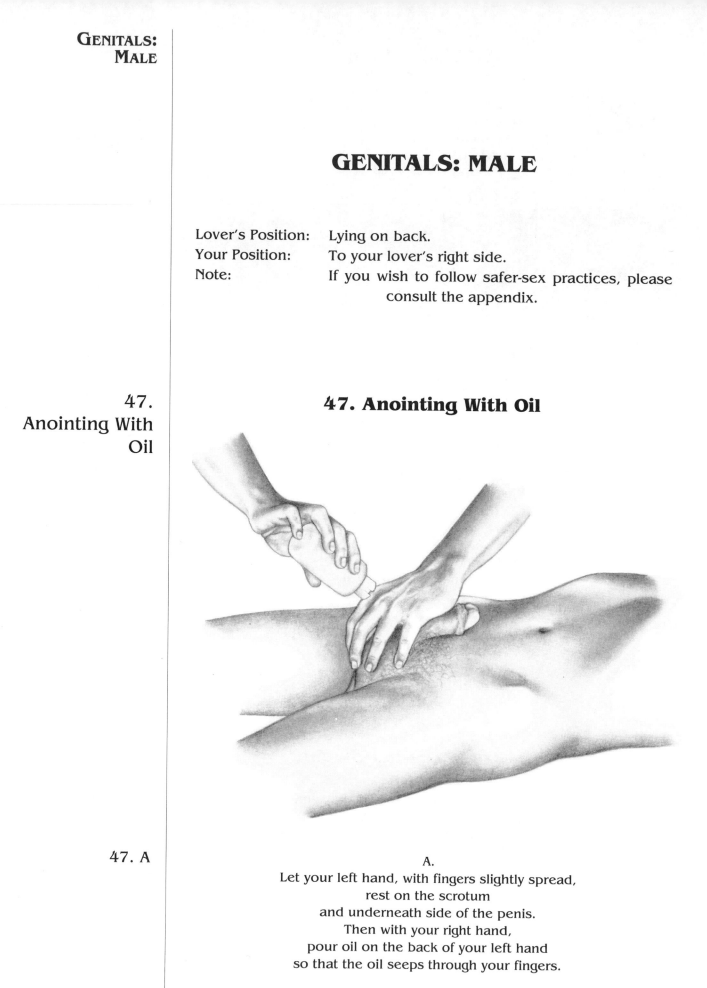

A.
Let your left hand, with fingers slightly spread,
rest on the scrotum
and underneath side of the penis.
Then with your right hand,
pour oil on the back of your left hand
so that the oil seeps through your fingers.

Anointing With
Oil

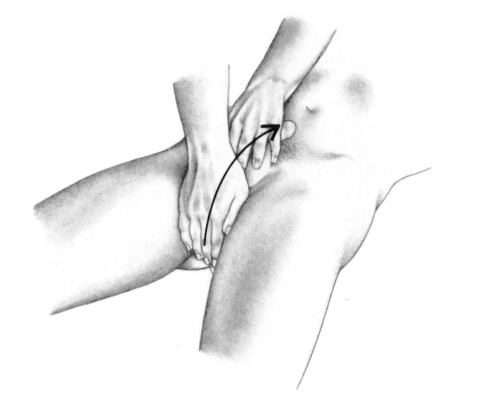

B.
Alternating your hands,
spread the oil with a pulling up motion,
sliding from the pelvic floor up
over the scrotum and penis.

Perhaps give a little firmer pressure
on the pelvic floor.

Be sure there is plenty of oil
since the following strokes
assume well-lubricated motions.

~

Note: Should your lover ejaculate during this or any other stroke
perhaps go to "Being," #58.

47. B

48.
The Coronal
Stroke

48. The Coronal Stroke

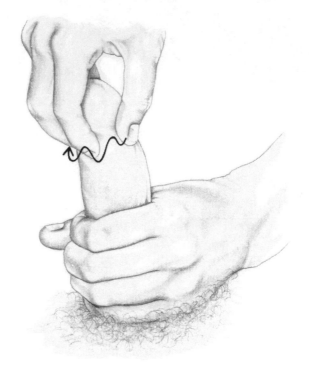

Your left hand gently stretches the foreskin down
along the shaft of the flaccid or erect penis.

Your right hand points
as if to twist a halved orange on a juicer.
Concentrating on the head of the penis,
rotate your right-hand fingers back and forth
in coordination with an up-and-down sliding motion.

Vary the amount of pressure from your right hand.

49. The Serpent

a: Your left hand gently stretches the foreskin down
along the shaft of the flaccid or erect penis.

Your right thumb and index finger form a snug circle
just below the head of the penis
and rotate in a clockwise direction
as far as your wrist permits.

49. a

b: Continuing the movement, lift your right thumb
so that your index finger can maintain
contact in the rotation
until the thumb can form a circle
with the index finger again.

~

Repeat this circling several times.

49. b

50. The Ten Stroke

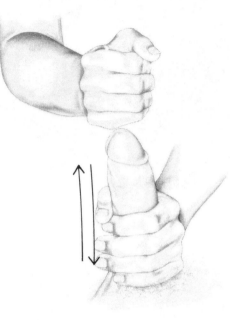

Using plenty of oil and alternating your hands,
make ten downward strokes
on the flaccid or erect penis,
then ten upward strokes.
Follow with nine downward, nine upward,
eight downward, eight upward
—all the way to one down and one up.

~

Suggestion:
syncopate the rhythm of your stroking.
Rather than using an even beat (1-2-3-4-5-6),
wait a moment after each set of two strokes
(1-2—3-4—5-6).

51. The Scrotum Ring

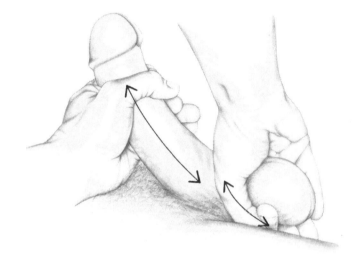

Your right thumb along with your index
and perhaps middle fingers
encircle the scrotum
between the base of the penis and the testicles.
(Be careful not to squeeze the testicles.)

Now move the scrotum up and down
as your left hand strokes up and down
on the flaccid or erect penile shaft.

Vary the amount of pressure of your right hand
against the base of the penis.

~

To continue the Male Genital strokes,
go to "Inner Connections," #57,
which is for both men and women.

GENITALS: FEMALE

Lover's Position: Lying on back.
Your Position: To your lover's right side.
Note: Be certain your fingernails are smooth and short
          and your hands are clean
          when massaging membranous tissues areas.
Note: If you wish to follow safer-sex practices,
          please consult the appendix.

52.
Anointing With
Oil

52. Anointing With Oil

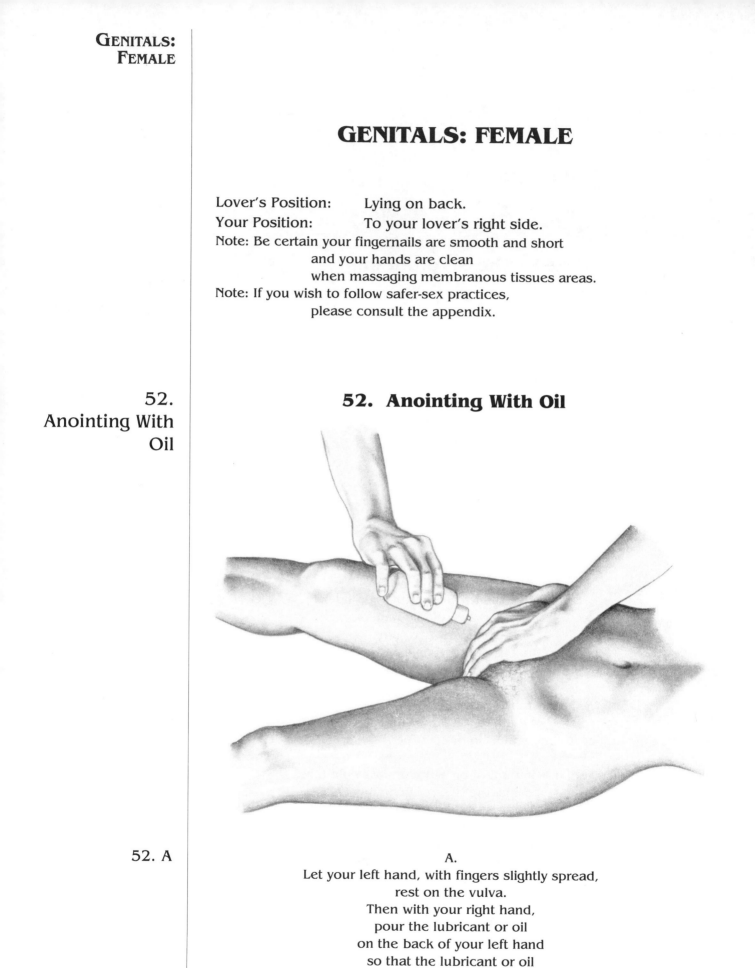

52. A

A.
Let your left hand, with fingers slightly spread,
rest on the vulva.
Then with your right hand,
pour the lubricant or oil
on the back of your left hand
so that the lubricant or oil
seeps through your fingers.

Anointing With
Oil

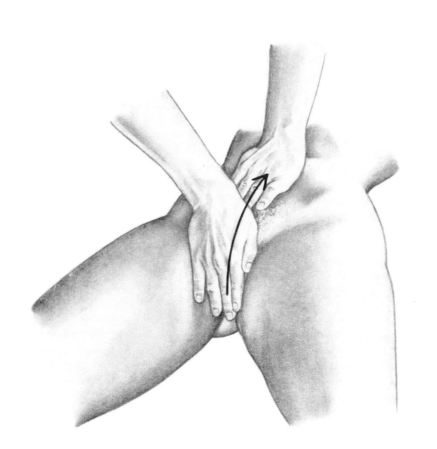

B.
Alternating your hands,
spread the lubricant or oil with a pulling up motion
by sliding from the lower part of the vulva
up over the clitoris and pubic area.

~

Note:
Be very careful not to stroke
from the anal to the vaginal areas.

52. B

53. The Vulva Stroke

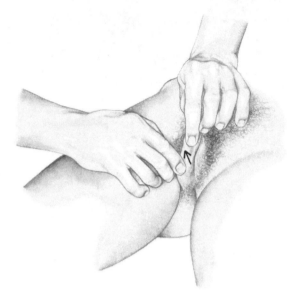

This is a series of strokes on each outer and inner lip.
With a thumb on one side of a lip
and the index finger on the other side,
very gently squeeze and slide off the edge of the lip.

Alternating your hands, continue this pattern
along the entire length of each lip.

54. The Clitoris Stroke

A.

Now you center your stroking
around the head of the clitoris,
which is just beneath where the inner lips
merge together at the upper part of the vulva.

To begin,
slide the middle finger pad of your right hand
up and down several times
between the inner and outer lips
on one side of the vulva
and then on the other side.

B.

With one or two fingers, slowly massage circles
around the clitoral head,
several times in one direction,
then several times in the other direction.

C.

With a single finger pad,
begin a very slow, upward stroke
at the vaginal entrance,
up through the inner lips, up past the clitoral head.
Repeat several times.

55.
The Clock

55. A

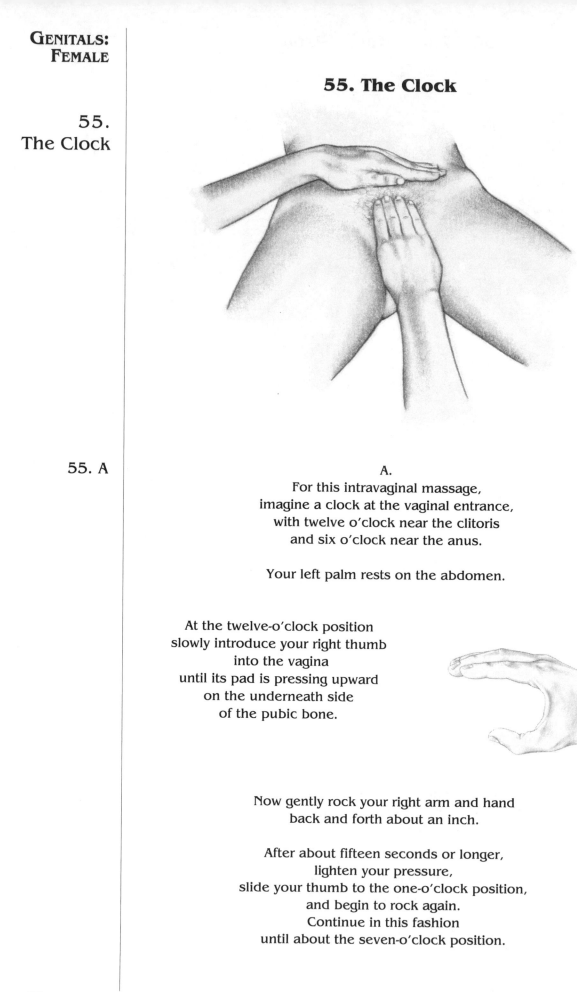

A.
For this intravaginal massage,
imagine a clock at the vaginal entrance,
with twelve o'clock near the clitoris
and six o'clock near the anus.

Your left palm rests on the abdomen.

At the twelve-o'clock position
slowly introduce your right thumb
into the vagina
until its pad is pressing upward
on the underneath side
of the pubic bone.

Now gently rock your right arm and hand
back and forth about an inch.

After about fifteen seconds or longer,
lighten your pressure,
slide your thumb to the one-o'clock position,
and begin to rock again.
Continue in this fashion
until about the seven-o'clock position.

The Clock

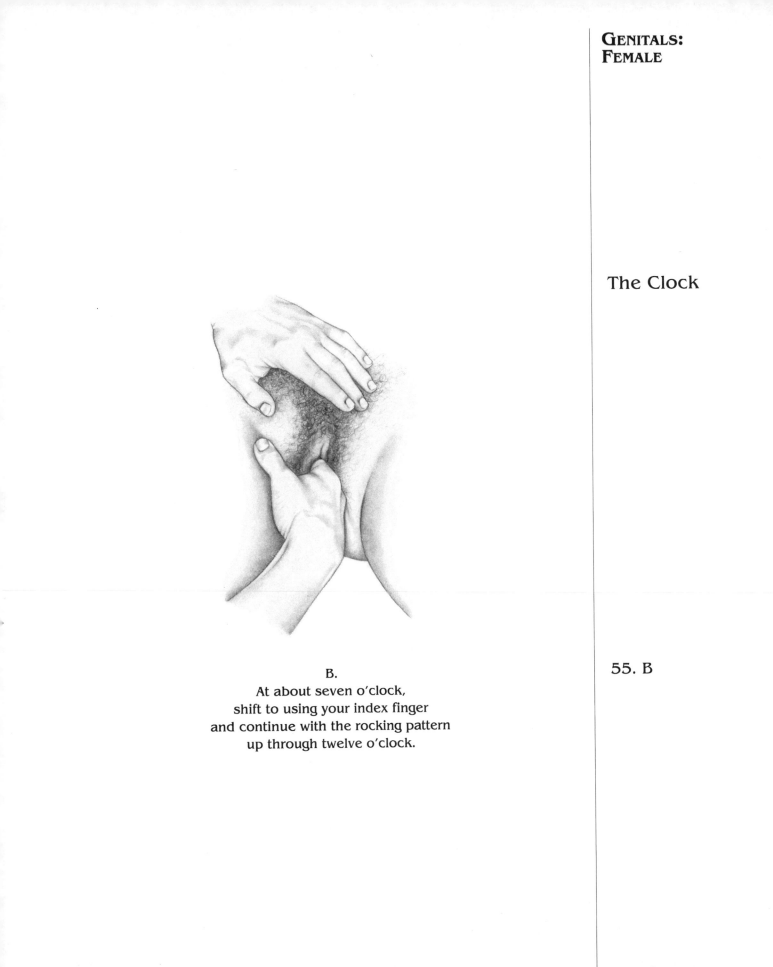

B.
At about seven o'clock,
shift to using your index finger
and continue with the rocking pattern
up through twelve o'clock.

55. B

GENITALS:
FEMALE

56.
The G-Spot
Stroke

56. A

56. The G-Spot Stroke

A.
This stroke may be easier
if you bring your lover's knees up
with both feet resting on the table.

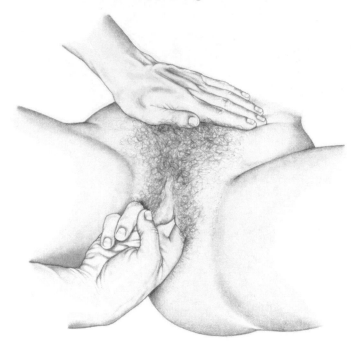

Your left palm rests on the abdomen.

At the twelve-o'clock position
slowly introduce
your right index and middle fingers
into the vagina
until the finger pads are pressing
upward
above (beyond) the pubic bone.
(This is approximately
the G-Spot area
inside the vagina.)

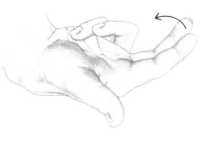

Here make a "come here" finger movement
to stroke your finger pads
across the membranous tissue.
Vary the pressure to find what feels best
— if there is pain,
lighten the pressure or discontinue the stroking.

The G-Spot
Stroke

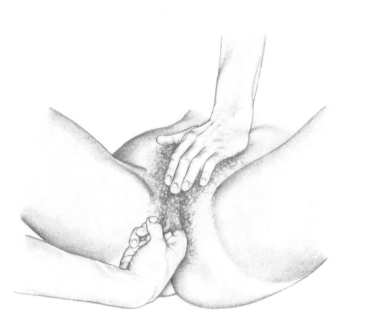

B.
With your right hand continuing Part A,
rest the heel of your left hand on the lower abdomen.
Now allow your left-hand fingers to delicately stroke the clitoral head
at the same time.

(Perhaps apply a little pressure
on the lower abdomen
with the heel of your left hand.)

When you complete the stroke,
slide your lover's legs back to the flat position.

56. B

Note: Starting with this stroke, the male and female genital massage description is the same.

57. Inner Connections

In this series of strokes
you connect the enjoyable sensations of the genitals
with the enjoyable sensations
of other parts of the body.

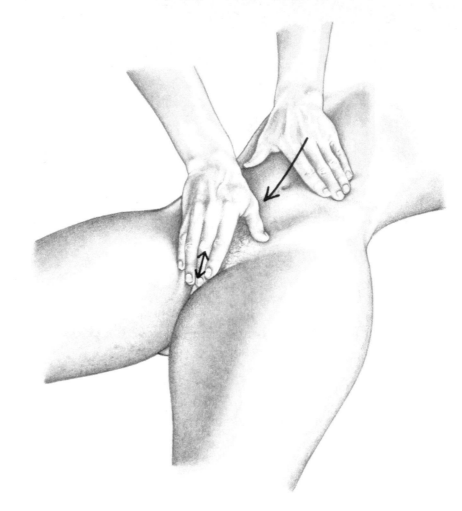

A. Abdomen and Genitals

While your right hand massages the genitals
(in any fashion)
let your left hand knead
or make circular strokes on the abdomen
(For a description of kneading, see stroke #9.)

Inner
Connections

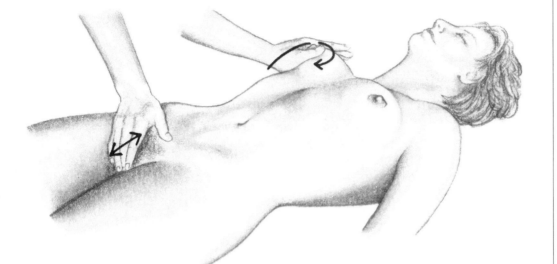

B. Breast Area and Genitals

57. B

As your right hand continues as in Part A,
slide your left hand from the same lower, outer side of the breast area
up over the breast
so that your thumb and index finger
encircle the nipple.
Using the nipple as the axis,
continue the stroke
by rotating your left hand clockwise
around the nipple
as you slide up and off the breast.
~
Repeat several times on the right breast area
and continue Part C on the right side of the neck
before going to the left side.

Inner
Connections

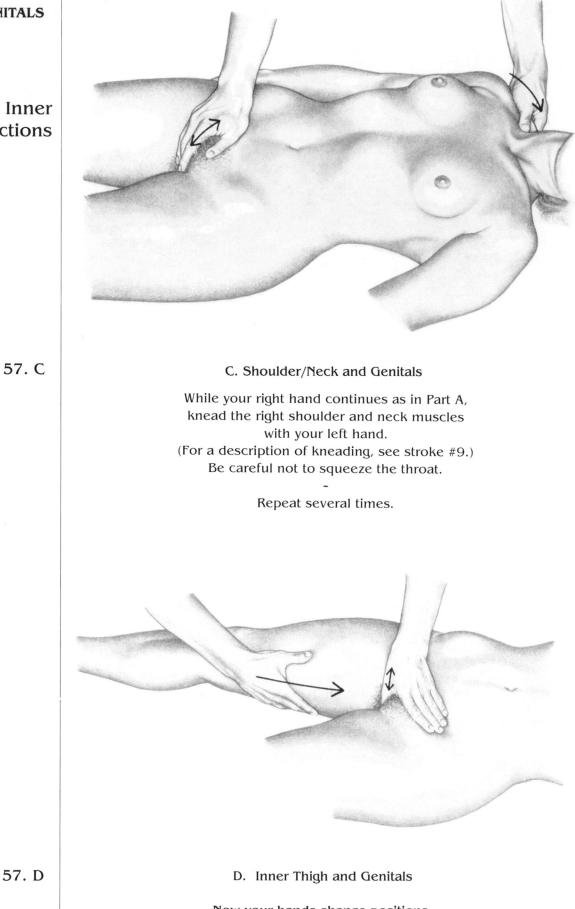

57. C

C. Shoulder/Neck and Genitals

While your right hand continues as in Part A,
knead the right shoulder and neck muscles
with your left hand.
(For a description of kneading, see stroke #9.)
Be careful not to squeeze the throat.

~

Repeat several times.

57. D

D. Inner Thigh and Genitals

Now your hands change positions:
your left sliding down to massage the genitals
while your right kneads the right inner thigh.

Inner
Connections

57. E

E. Change Sides

If it is possible, move to the other side
and follow the same sequence
while simply reversing
the left-hand and right-hand instructions.
(If you cannot easily move to the over side,
modify your stroking so that the left breast,
neck/shoulder, and thigh areas are massaged also.)

Once you complete this series,
move back to your lover's right side
for the following instructions.
(Remember to keep hand contact if possible.)

58.
Being

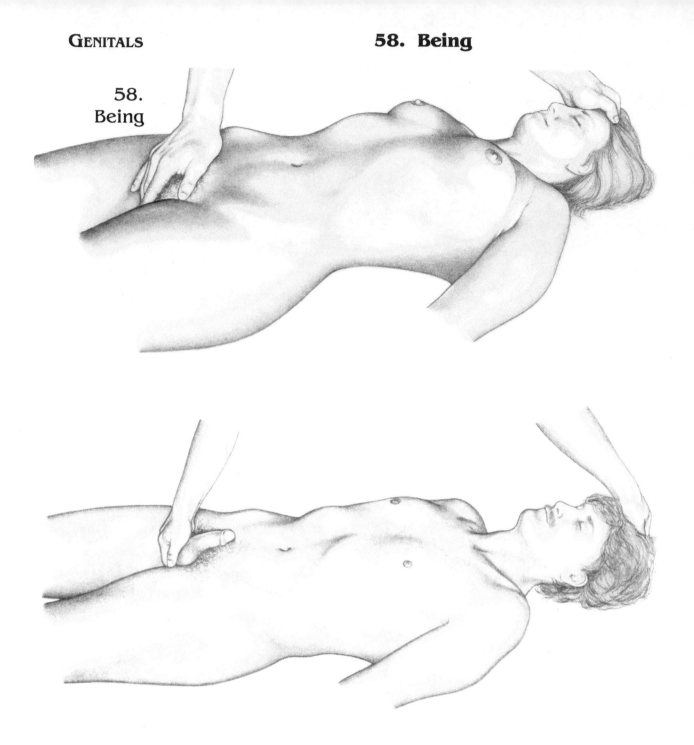

58. A

A.
Rest your left hand on the head
so that your palm is on the forehead
and your fingers are on the center top of the head.

At the other end of an imaginary axis
through the core of the body,
rest your right hand on the pelvic area
so that your palm is on the vulva,
or the scrotum if you are massaging a man.

(58. A continued)

Now give a soft verbal invitation to your beloved
to take a slightly fuller inhalation
and to imagine the breath
beginning at the floor of his/her pelvis
and coming up the core of the body
to the top of his/her head.

Then for the exhalation,
invite your beloved to simply let go of the breath
and to imagine the breath reversing
and flowing from the top of the head
down through the core of the body
and out the floor of the pelvis.

~

Continue this breathing and imaging guidance
for perhaps two to five minutes.

~

Here we are focusing directly
on the subtle energy bodies.
In the pelvic floor area is
the first, or Muladhara, chakra.
At the top of the head is
the crown, or Sahasrara, chakra.

Often the genital massage
stimulates sexual feelings,
turns on the generator in the pelvic area.
This laying on of hands, Being,
encourages the expansion of energy
throughout the body.

This is the shift
from friction sex
to tantric sex.

Being

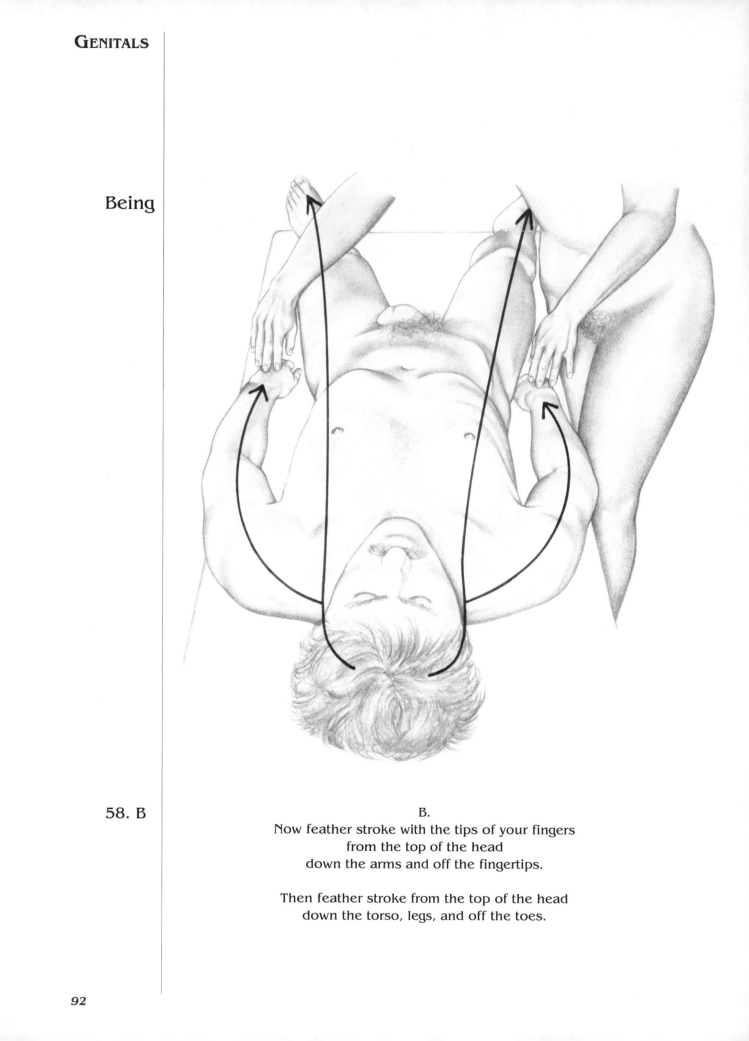

58. B

B.
Now feather stroke with the tips of your fingers
from the top of the head
down the arms and off the fingertips.

Then feather stroke from the top of the head
down the torso, legs, and off the toes.

Being

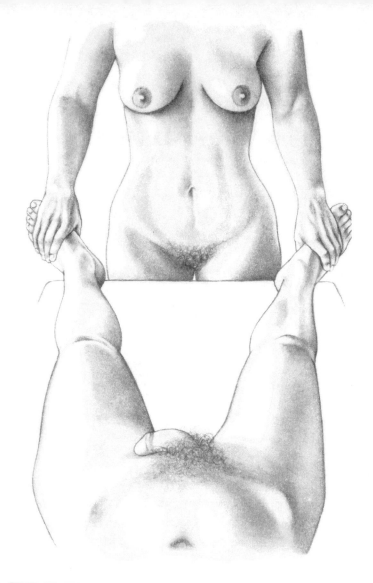

58. C

C.
Now rest your hands on the feet
with your thumbs on the arches
and your fingers on top of the feet.

Here again softly give breathing
and imaging instructions:
the inhalation comes from the bottom of the feet
up to the top of the head
The exhalation flows from the top of the head
down to the bottom of the feet.

After a couple of minutes
gradually allow your hands to ascend,
up off your beloved's feet.

NECK AND HEAD

Your Position: Behind the head.

59. Connecting Stroke

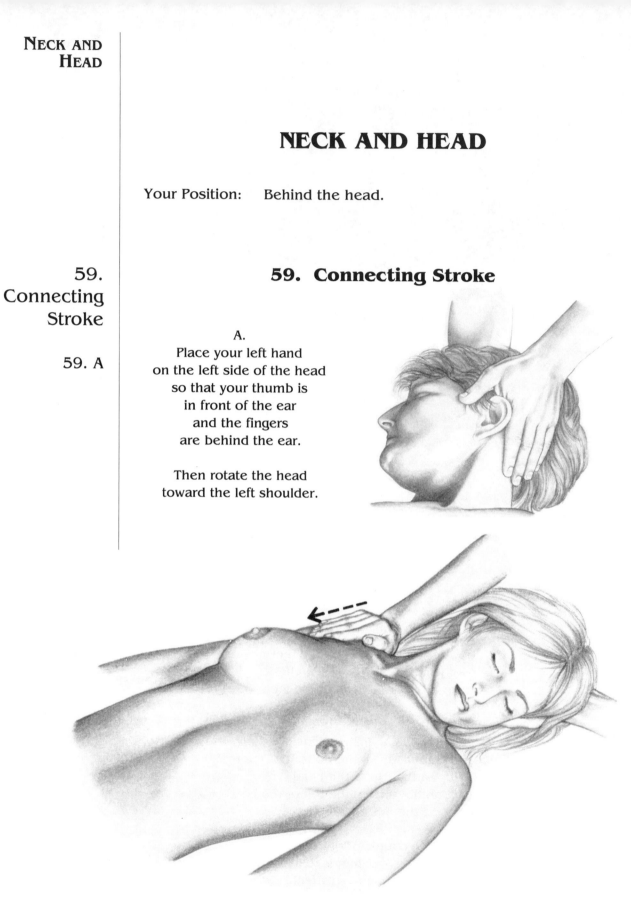

A.
Place your left hand
on the left side of the head
so that your thumb is
in front of the ear
and the fingers
are behind the ear.

Then rotate the head
toward the left shoulder.

B.
Place your right palm on the right shoulder
and stretch downward.

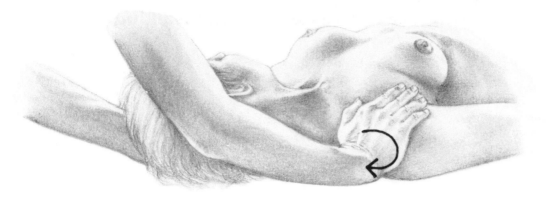

C.
Discontinue the stretching
and pivot your hand outward on the shoulder.

D.
Firmly slide the flat of your fingers upward
on the back of the neck
(not on the throat).

~

Repeat steps B, C, and D several times
and then follow the same sequence
on the other side of the neck,
reversing the instructions
for your right and left hands.

60. Let The Fingers Do The Walking

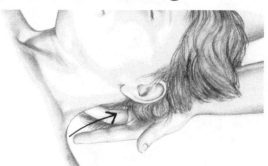

60.
Let The
Fingers Do The
Walking

With the head resting on
the heels of your palms,
"walk" the finger pads
upward
on the back of the neck.

The "walking" is a sliding movement
of alternating fingers
from the base of the neck
toward the bottom of the skull.
(Use a firm pressure with your fingers,
but be careful not to pull the hair.)

61.
Head Scratch

61. Head Scratch

61. A

A.
Slide your finger pads back and forth
across the scalp on the underneath side of the head.

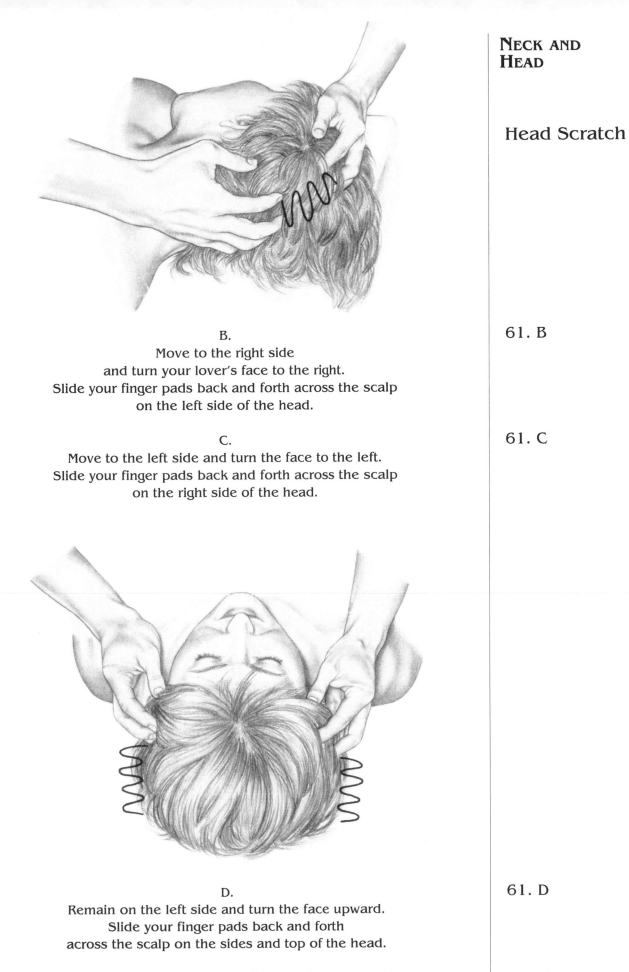

Head Scratch

B.
Move to the right side
and turn your lover's face to the right.
Slide your finger pads back and forth across the scalp
on the left side of the head.

61. B

C.
Move to the left side and turn the face to the left.
Slide your finger pads back and forth across the scalp
on the right side of the head.

61. C

D.
Remain on the left side and turn the face upward.
Slide your finger pads back and forth
across the scalp on the sides and top of the head.

Gradually quicken the speed (but not the pressure).

61. D

Tantric Massage

E.
Without slowing down,
suddenly lift your fingers off the head.

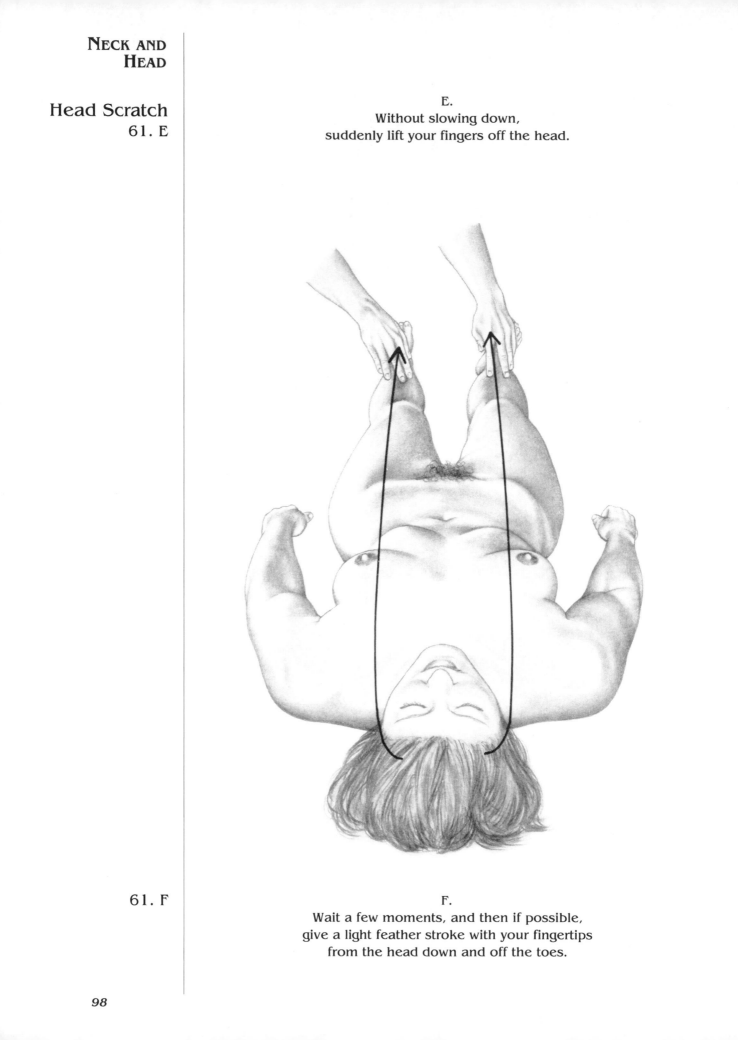

61. F

F.
Wait a few moments, and then if possible,
give a light feather stroke with your fingertips
from the head down and off the toes.

FACE

Your Position: Behind the head.

Note: It is best not to apply more oil for a facial massage. However, if you have been using an unscented oil, you might try a small drop of scented oil.

62. T Stroke

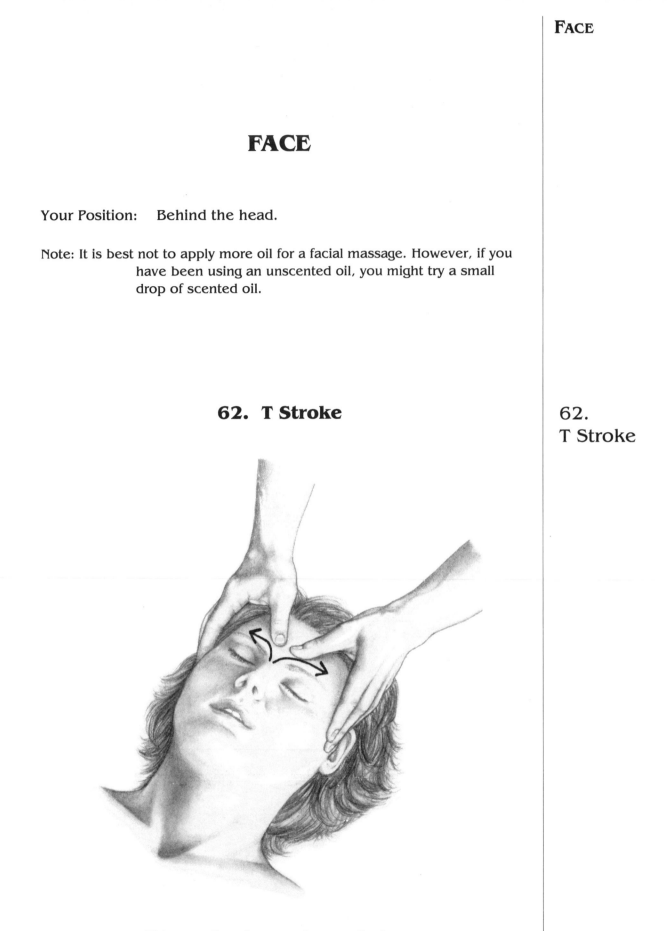

Slide your thumbs up and across the brow.
Three or four repetitions
will probably cover the whole brow.

63. Eyebrow Squeeze

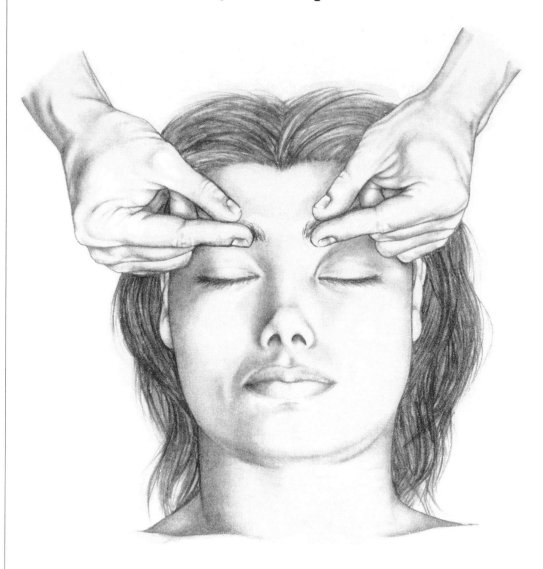

Make a series of squeezes of the eyebrows
from the midline outward.

64. Temple Circles

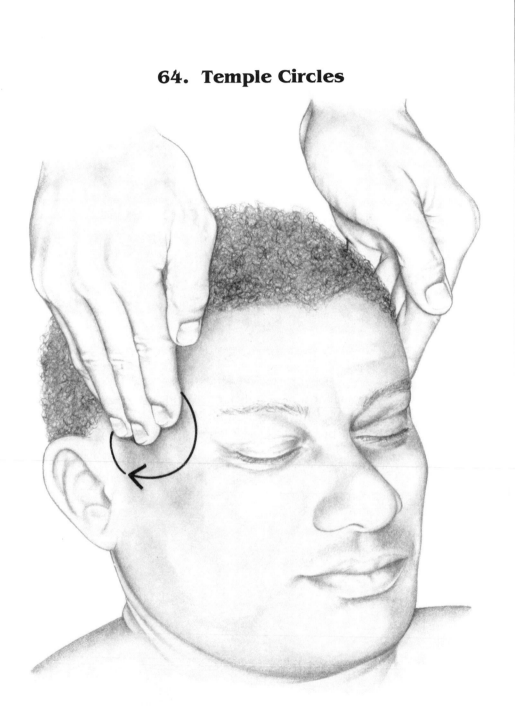

Make circle movements on the temples
with flat fingers.
Apply enough pressure
so his/her skin slides over the muscles beneath.

65. Underneath-The-Eyes Stroke

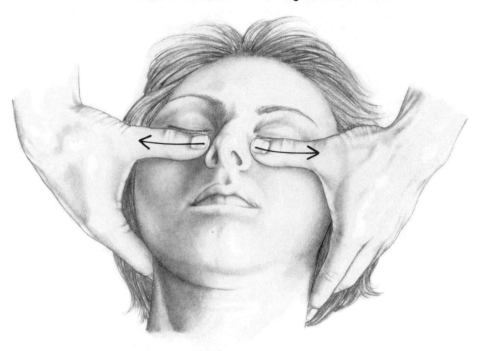

Slide your thumbs outward across the bony surface
underneath the eyes.

66. Eye Stroke

Massage the eyes only if hard contact lens
have been removed;
light pressure on soft lens may be OK.

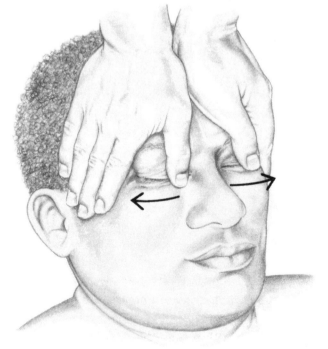

Bracing the heel of your thumbs on the forehead,
slowly slide your thumb pads
outward across the closed eyes.
Repeat two or three times.

67. Cheek Bone Stroke

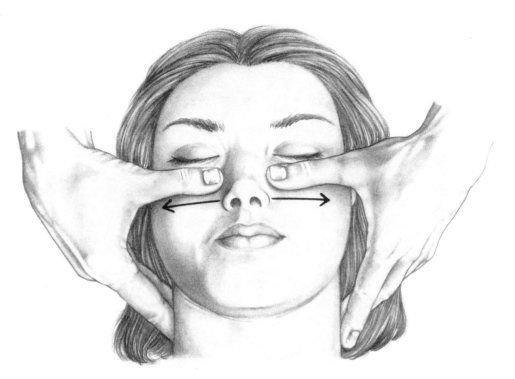

Slide your thumbs outward
across the top of the cheek bone.

68. Under-The-Cheek-Bone Stroke

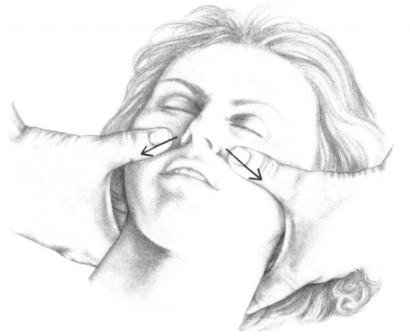

Slide your thumbs outward
underneath the cheek bone.

69.
Jaw Circles

69. Jaw Circles

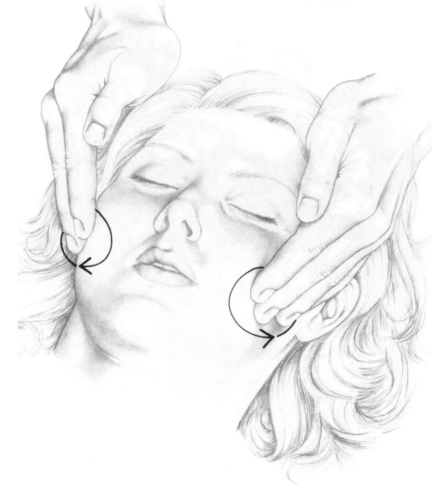

Make circle movements on the jaw area
with flat fingers.
Apply enough pressure
so his/her skin slides over the muscles beneath.

70.
Upper Lip
Stroke

70. Upper Lip Stroke

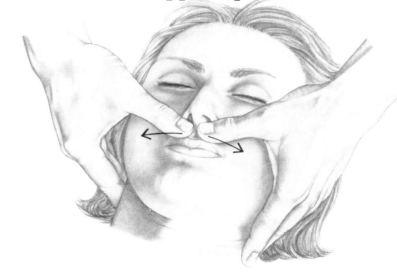

Slide your thumbs outward across the upper lip.

71. Lower Lip Stroke

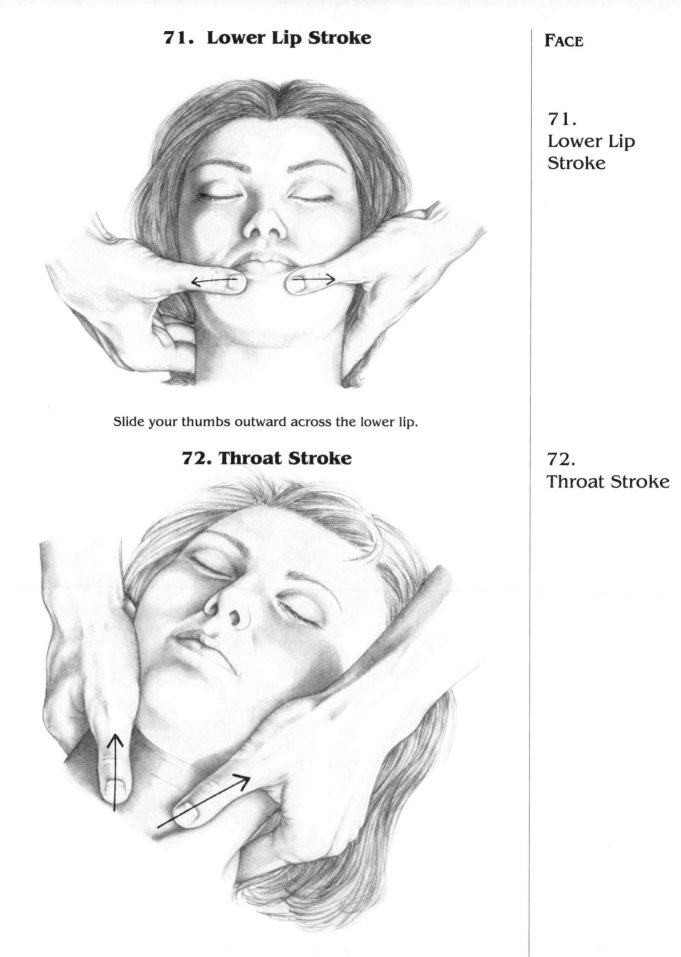

Slide your thumbs outward across the lower lip.

72. Throat Stroke

Slide your thumbs upward along the groove
between the larynx and the sides of the throat.

73. Behind-The-Ear Stroke

73.
Behind-The-Ear
Stroke

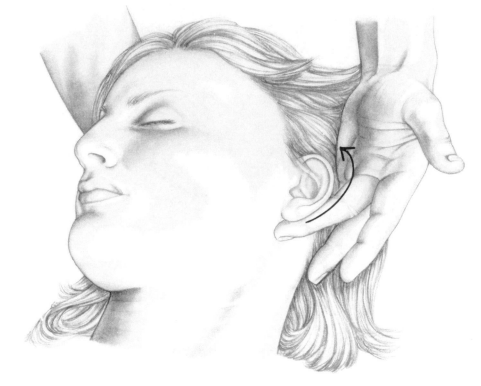

Slide your middle fingers
up and down along the grooves
behind the ears.

74.
Outer Ear
Stroke

74. Outer Ear Stroke

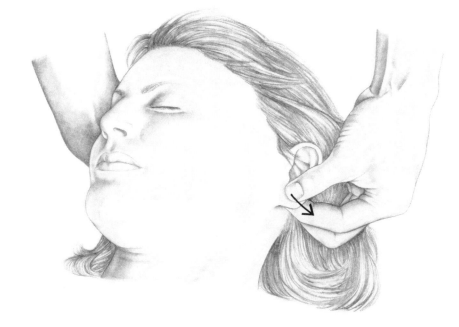

Gently squeeze the ear lobes
and slide outward to the edges.

~

Repeat this along the entire outer ear surface.

75. Inner Peace

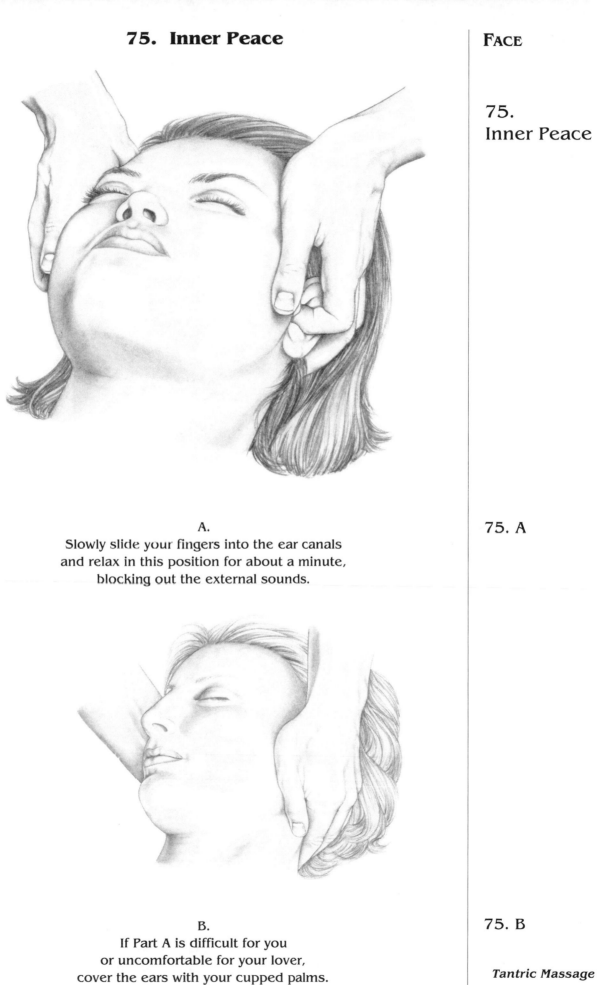

A.
Slowly slide your fingers into the ear canals
and relax in this position for about a minute,
blocking out the external sounds.

75. A

B.
If Part A is difficult for you
or uncomfortable for your lover,
cover the ears with your cupped palms.

75. B

76.
Concluding
Stroke

77.
Covering

CONCLUSION

76. Concluding Stroke

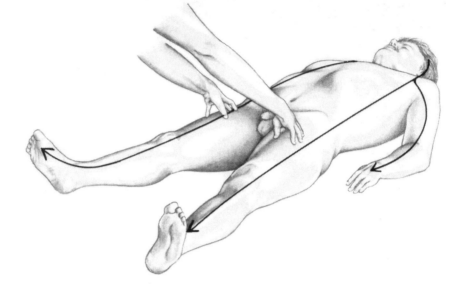

With your fingertips,
lightly feather stroke from the top of the head
down off the fingertips.
Then lightly feather stroke from the top of the head
down off the toes.

77. Covering

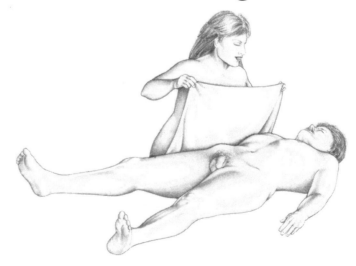

Unless it is very warm,
cover your beloved with a towel or sheet.

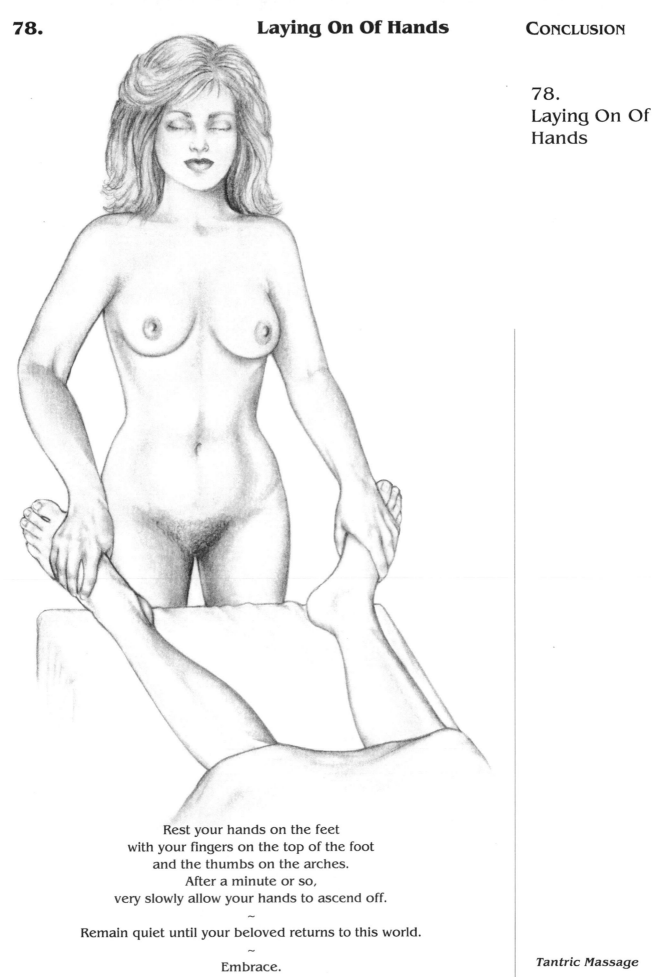

Rest your hands on the feet
with your fingers on the top of the foot
and the thumbs on the arches.
After a minute or so,
very slowly allow your hands to ascend off.

~

Remain quiet until your beloved returns to this world.

~

Embrace.

APPENDIX

Eroticizing Safer Sex

Massage in general
     is considered in AIDS safer sex guidelines
     to be a no-risk or very-low-risk activity.

When there is uncertainty
     about the giver's or receiver's health
     or if either partner is communicable
     with the AIDS virus,
          you may wish to read the following.

Current research indicates that
     when blood, ejaculate, or vaginal lubrications
     come in contact
     with a broken skin or membranous tissue surface,
     the transmission risk may increase.

Should you prefer to follow AIDS safer sex practices
     when massaging the male or female genital area,
     it is recommended
     to wear latex or vinyl examination gloves,
     which you can purchase at a pharmacy
          or surgical supply store.

(Concerning infectious skin conditions,
     such as herpes lesions or venereal warts,
     it is recommended to entirely forego contact
     with the communicable area
          or to consult a medical professional.)

When using a latex product,
     apply only a water-based lubricant
          since oil can deteriorate latex.
     If the water-based lubricant contains nonoxynol-9,
     which can destroy the AIDS virus on contact,
     the protection will be supplemented.
     Some people, though, are sensitive to nonoxynol-9.

An alternative or an addition to wearing gloves
        in a male genital massage
        is to place a condom on the penis.
Try a few drops of water-based lubricant
        in the tip of the condom before unrolling it.
Some of the strokes in this book, however,
        are best suited for gloves without a condom.

At first, these protective measures
        might appear as intrusions or hindrances.
After exploration, you may find,
        as many others have,
that latex and vinyl examination gloves
provide some uniquely smooth sensations,
that the water-based lubricant inside the condom
creates heretofore unexperienced pleasures.

Eroticizing safer sex means
        letting go of expectations
        and allowing the discovery of new worlds.
Giving the touch of love,
        as in the sensual massage offered in this book,
        can bring us all closer
        to these new worlds of pleasure.

ACKNOWLEDGMENTS

Louise-Andrée Saulnier was the collaborator in the first edition of this book. It was through her love, support, and encouragement that I was to write and publish this first book to illustrate genital massage explicitly, a project no other publisher was willing to touch. I greatly appreciate her.

My principal meditation teachers, Tarthang Tulku and Billie Hobart, were a major influence on this book though they taught little about massage or sexuality.

The underlying massage style in *Tantric Massage* evolved in the early days of humanistic psychology. I wish to express my gratitude to Margaret Elke, whose work in massage and sensuality has influenced many, and to the pioneering teachers at Esalen Institute.

The students and faculty of The Institute for Advanced Study of Human Sexuality in San Francisco have continuously supported my teaching massage as a means to bring the sensual and intimate qualities into the sexual expression.

I am indebted to Clark Taylor, Ph.D., and David Lourea, Ed.D., of the Sexologists' Sexual Health Project in San Francisco for their support in eroticizing safer sex. I am equally thankful to Molly Hogan, R.N., Norma Wilcox, R.N., and Sharon Miller, M.S.

Finding an artist with both the sensitivity and the willingness to illustrate the subject matter of this book was a major undertaking. The sensual, spiritual eroticism of Kyle Spencer graces the pages of *Tantric Massage.* Her abilities and expressions inspire me.

My dear friend, Ellen Gunther, M.D., provided the photography on which the massage technique illustrations were based.

I greatly appreciate the support from so many others in so many ways: Chris McMahon, Chyrelle D. Chasen, Clara Kerns, Joseph Kramer, Lynn Craig, Mary Jane Harper, Nora LaCorte, Pam Johnson, Sandy Trupp, Saunya Tolson, Vicki Folz, Wendell Lipscomb, as well as others.

EPILOGUE

My beloved is gone down into his garden,
to the beds of spices,
to feed in the gardens,
and to gather lilies.

I am my beloved's,
and my beloved is mind:
he feedeth among the lilies.

The Song of Solomon 6:2-3

This is the touch of love.

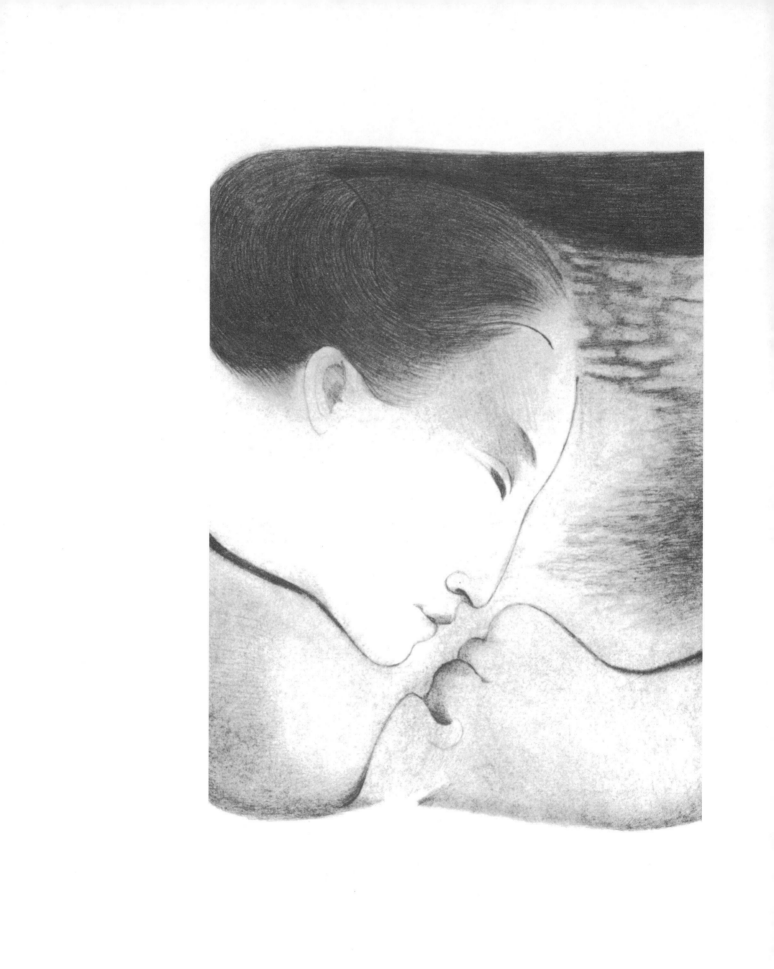

Sensual Ceremony

Dedicated to
Sun Dancer
Fly free, my friend.

ACKNOWLEDGMENTS

Sensual Ceremony evolved out of my experience of giving over three hundred Secret Garden ceremonies to friends, lovers, and strangers-becoming-friends. These people and ceremonies are special moments in my life.

The Secret Garden Ceremony might never have evolved were it not for Sun Dancer. He was the catalyst when the ceremony was only in my imagination. His friendship is both precious and auspicious for me.

Without Chyrelle D. Chasen this manuscript might have sat in storage another ten years. Thank you so much for your loving support.

Richard Stodart, the illustrator, embodies a sensual spirit in his heart. I feel blessed.

Sandy Trupp, friend and publishing advisor, is always an inspiration.

There are many others to whom I am deeply grateful: Bettina Suppe, Carole Merette, Clara Kerns, and Pam Johnson.

PREFACE

Traditionally, massage is usually taught as technique. After I learned the technique, I discovered more. When approached with a mindfulness of and the honoring of the wholeness of another, massage is a ceremony.

Sensual Ceremony is my evolution of my massage as I allowed many nuances and embellishments to unfold. The following are many possibilities amongst many ways to sensually celebrate and commune with another.

There is one additional point I wish to emphasize. Massaging another's mind with guided imagery, as in Chapter 4, can be a far more powerful method than we might think. In such guided experiences, we invite the recipient to sense all the different types of physical senses but in inner space. Here the recipient sees, touches, smells, tastes, and hears in a different dimension.

The objective in these guided imageries is to discover whatever is revealed. Here it is very important not to attempt to influence what the recipient is to do or to feel when back in everyday consciousness. Our inner self can be a wiser guide. So at least when doing the ceremonies that follow, refrain from suggestions for after the guided imagery. Allow the inner self to dance, to sing, to teach as it wishes throughout the ceremony.

This is, in fact, the guideline for the whole sensual ceremony. Allow the recipient's soul to soar with its own wisdom. As the giver, we will be blessed by the inner beauty that blossoms before our eyes—and hands.

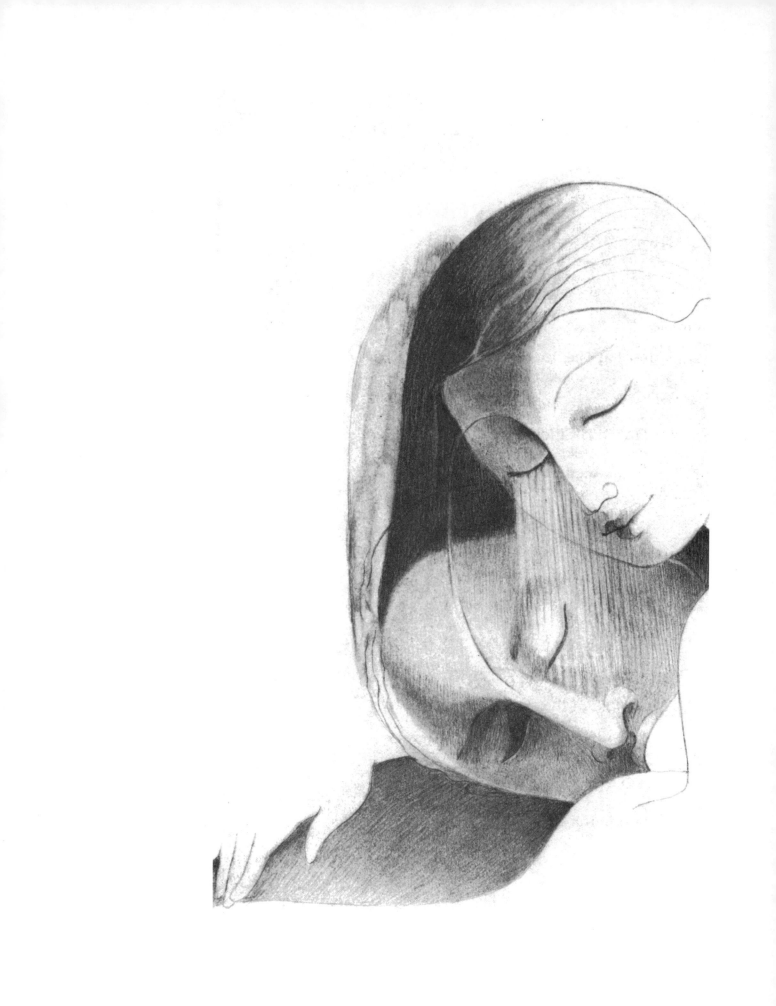

INVITATION

A candle flame radiating

A finger resting

A peacock feather caressing

A mango melting

A stream of warm water searching

Arms embracing

Becoming One

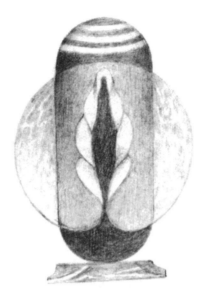

INTRODUCTION

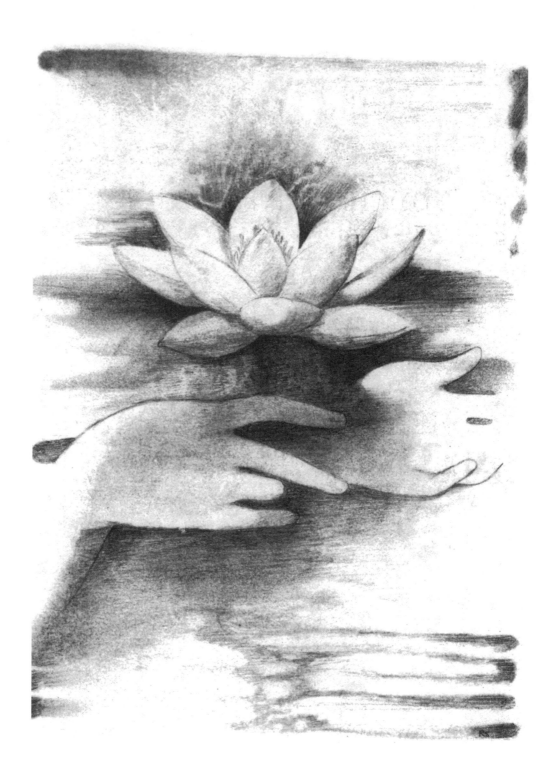

1 Touching The Heart
Ceremonial Sensual Pleasuring

Ceremony is presence
>It is being
>>rather than doing or having
>It is attentive awareness

Ceremony is purposeful spontaneity
>It is flowing pattern
>It is simple elegance

A ceremony is not
>a mindless routine
>>though many ceremonial structures
>>have become this
>A ceremony can be
>>in solitude
>>with another
>>or with many others
>There is a conscious beginning and ending

In ceremony
>there is a sense
>>of wholeness
>>of connection
>>of communion

In sensual ceremony
>we embrace the senses
>>through presence
>>through ambiance

through touch
taste
fragrance
tone and timbre
color and form

A sensual ceremony is a special gift
It is a physical sharing
of warmth and caring
It is an expression of tenderness
Giving this gift of pleasure
we invite another
to be guided into the inner garden
Here, in the quiet of sanctuary
we nourish each sense
Here, the inner flower
awakens and blooms

Our softly spoken words
weave a meadow
In herbal waters
we bathe
Our fingers
squeeze drops of sweetness
from fresh fruit
Lullabying,
we embrace
Like island breezes
we caress with feathers
Glistening with oil
our hands dance

When each sense
is nurtured in gentleness
the heart is touched
and we experience joy
This is the underlying philosophy

ASCETICISM, HEDONISM, TANTRA

Generally there are two orientations
toward the body and the senses:
the ascetic and the hedonistic

The ascetic philosophy
views anything that is
pleasing to the senses

as obstructive/destructive
to human development
either in material or spiritual attainment
There can be
abstention / denial / sometimes self-inflicted discomfort
The accompanying attitude
may be one of
condescension or disgust
toward the body
The implication,
pleasures of the flesh
lack meaningfulness,
they are addictive,
there is no real contribution
to the individual and society
The assumption,
there is something
inherently negative/evil about the body
After yielding to temptation
one must seek atonement

At the opposite end,
the hedonistic philosophy
Here one intensely pursues
gratification of desires
There is a grasping attempt
to hoard/consume

There is a story
about how a monkey can be captured
The end of a coconut
is cut off
and a handful of rice placed inside
Finding the prize
the monkey reaches inside
to grasp the rice
However, to get the fist back through
the narrow opening,
the hand must first relax
and let go of the rice
Unwilling to cease its grasping,
the monkey becomes burdened
and is easily captured

It is as if
there are strings of attachment
binding a hedonist
to a desired object
Without continued titillation
life becomes boring

Pointing a finger at such behavior
     an ascetic would label a hedonist
        indulgent / decadent / narcissistic

There is another path, *tantra*
    This philosophy
        neither damns nor craves
           the body and the sense experiences
    Rather than being obstacles,
        the sensations/feelings
        become the vehicles of self-realization and well-being

Tantra
        a Sanskrit word
    comes to us from some schools
        of Buddhism and Hinduism
    Translated sometimes from a derivation of *to weave*
        sometimes a combination of
           to expand and *to liberate*
    Acceptance
        is a central teaching
    Embracing the sensory experiences,
           surrendering consciously to the moment
        we transcend
           the world of attachment
    Allowing the flow of feelings
        we develop empathy
        deepen intimacy
    Our mindfulness, our meditations
        transform the energies
           of each experience,
        liberating us
           from the limitations of grasping and avoiding

Here we open ourself
        to a reverence for beauty
    An aesthetic appreciation
        enriches the meaning of life
In tantra
    we celebrate
        the heart and the senses
In tantra
    we are
        at-one-ment

2 Kissing The Joy As It Flies
Giving The Gift

TRUST GUIDELINES

A sensual ceremony
        is for anyone in our life
                female or male
                friend or lover
        for whom we wish
        to express our love

Simply present an invitation
        Be open to receiving "no"

Communicate
                verbally or nonverbally
                explicitly or implicitly
        the following guidelines

1.   "If there is anything I am doing or providing
                        that you want more of,
                let me know"
2.   "If there is anything I am doing or providing
                        that is either uncomfortable or undesirable,
                let me know"
3.   "If there is anything that I am not doing or providing
                        that you want,
                let me know"
4.   "Regarding your requests,
                if I am willing and able to fulfill them,

I will do so
If I am either unwilling or unable to,
I will let you know"
(Though the intention
in most of the sensual ceremonies here
is for the recipient to receive without giving back,
this is open to renegotiation)

5.   "As much as possible,
allow yourself to experience
your sensations and your feelings"

Following these guidelines
means that both the giver and receiver
have choice
From freedom of choice,
joy and love flow
Having, making, and communicating choices
are the cornerstone of trust

THE FOUR LIMITATIONS

There are four psychological patterns
that can limit sensual ceremony

Spectatoring/Performing

If we keep our attention on
"Am I doing it right?" or "wrong?"
we are like a spectator
watching for a flaw in a performance on a stage
Our mind has a standard
that we have to live up to
When we are in this state
there is limited spontaneity and pleasure
Our awareness is on *should*
rather than our sensations and feelings

Judgments of Others

A judgment
    is a perspective
        that something a person is, does, or has
            is not all right with me
    Something is not OK
        by my standard
    Another is
        too short
        too fat
        too rich
        late too often
        eats the wrong food
        leaves the cap off the toothpaste...
    We can have intimacy
        to the extent
            that we are willing to let go of our judgments
        to the extent
            we allow a person
            to be exactly the way she/he is
                and is not

Comparisons with the Past

In our mind
    we can stretch a special moment into hours
        make the sensations vibrant
        deepen the profoundness of tender emotions
    Reliving feelings
        by remembering the events of the past
            can be meaningful and beautiful

We rob ourself, however,
        when we try to superimpose
        the past on the present
    We often find
        the present does not live up to
        that special event in the past
    If we use the images from the past
        to invalidate the present
        we experience
            neither value nor beauty

Expectations of the Future

When we have a standard
aimed at the future
we term it *expectation*
In our anticipation
we usually miss what is happening
in the moment
And then when the future arrives
and does not fulfill our expectations
our attention goes to what is lacking
In our emotional upset
we again miss the richness
of what is available
to our senses in the present

Letting Go

The extent to which
we can let go
of these limitations
is the extent to which
we can have pleasure in our life
Here are three suggestions

First, we can acknowledge
that we are the source of our
spectatoring/judgments/comparisons/expectations
Placing a cause elsewhere
we divert ourself
from the sensations/feelings
of the present
A second suggestion
is to not judge or reprimand ourself
Alternatively, we could view the situation as
an opportunity to learn about ourselves

Thirdly, enter a pleasuring activity
as ceremony
Perhaps attune yourself to the following teachings

TANTRIC TEACHINGS

To create a sense of ceremony,
        we can be mindful of
            receptivity
            relaxation response
            present-time experience

Receptivity means
        there is no attachment
            to the outcome of actions
Applying to both giving and receiving roles
        this quality emphasizes
            nonperformance and nondemand
On the surface
        receptivity may appear
            to be the same as passivity
To the contrary,
        receptivity requires
            awareness
            choice
        It is very different
            than *giving up*
            than nonchoice submissiveness
While receptivity emphasizes nonattachment
        there is no opposition to
            goals/directions
Were we to effort
        to achieve a desired outcome, however,
            we would blind ourself to many experiences
Efforting is opposite
        to the nature of ceremony
Allowing, rather than striving,
        is the key

Relaxation response means
        there is a relatively calm body/mind
This is in contrast
        to what we commonly call the fight-or-flight response
        When we are being chased by a hungry tiger
            we are not likely
            to be conscious
                of the jungle flowers' lovely fragrances
Physiologically speaking
        performance anxiety and striving
            create similar stress responses
        as fleeing from the tiger
If we are to truly appreciate the senses

we must have an inner calm

Present-time experience means
 we are not caught up
  in our expectations of the future
  or comparisons with the past
 To experience pleasure
  our attention must be in the present
 This quality by no means suggests
  that we deny or resist
   our comparisons or expectations
 Quite the contrary
  with all comparisons and expectations
   there are inner feeling experiences
    which also include body sensations
 In meditation
  these sensations
   can serve as attention focuses
 To place our awareness in our sensations
  is perhaps
   the most powerful method
  for coming back to present time,
   for being present

The three qualities
 receptivity, relaxation response, present-time experience
  are essential facets
 of ceremonial sensual pleasuring
When we *lose our senses*
 or fail to appreciate our universe
  these qualities can serve as signposts
  to the tantric path

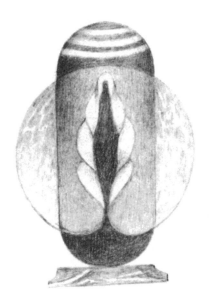

The Secret Garden Ceremony

If you wish to give a special gift
                    to express your love
                    to share communion
            explore the Secret Garden Ceremony
                    Here one *gives*
                            while another *receives*
            Similar to ancient tantric sexual rituals
                    in some ways,
                    the forms in this contemporary ceremony
                            may be more suitable
                            for many of us raised in Western culture

The following chapters present
                    the basic elements of
                            the Secret Garden Ceremony
            guided imagery
            feeding in the bath
            bathing
            massaging

Modify any part
                    according to your talents and desires
            You may prefer
                    to make an element
                            a whole ceremony in itself
            A sensual ceremony
                            may be for a few minutes
                            or several hours
                                    Duration is not the essence

Many specific details follow
                    based on much trial and error
                    based on many sensual ceremonies
            Allow the details
                    to serve you
                            when the information is relevant
            Attachment to details
                    limits spontaneity
                    constricts the expression of essence
            Nonattentiveness to details, however,
                    can result in nonceremony
It's a delicate balance

You may mutually choose
                    with your partner
            to be sexual, to be orgasmic
                            or not
                    before, during, or after
                            the ceremony

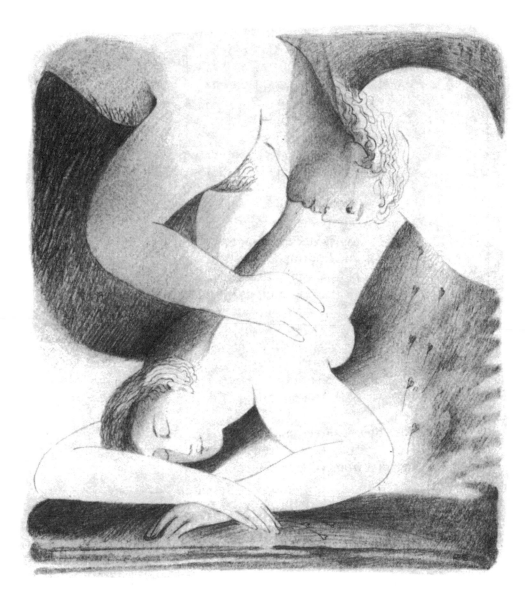

Enter the experience, however,
            without predetermined goals
    Allow each moment
                each feeling
        to unfold
                without attachment
        This is the tantric meditation

Overview

A few days prior to the Secret Garden Ceremony
        have a pre-interview
                with the recipient
    This may be unnecessary
            when giving to an intimate partner
                if you already know
                        the likes/dislikes
                        possible food and skin allergies
    The preinterview is a time
            to ask about feelings
            and to arrange logistics:
                    schedules, baby sitter
                    roommates out of the apartment
                    no obligations afterward...

If this gift
        is to be a surprise
                make sure the recipient has
                at least eight hours of unscheduled time

A few days before the ceremony
                shop for the fruit
    Market fruits often are insufficiently ripe

Anticipate at least one hour, possibly two or three
        for the preparation immediately prior
                to an extensive ceremony
        the Secret Garden Ceremony itself, if given in total
                could be three to six hours
    First, the guided imagery
            to calm the body/mind
            to discover the inner garden
            to create sanctuary
    Following, in the bath
            you nourish with fruits and sparkling nectar
                    in sensual communion

Next you bathe
in ceremonial waters
Then, anointing the temple of the spirit with oil
your hands massage
your beloved
Afterwards you might cuddle together
and breathe in unison
for another hour

A few days later
you might reflect together
sharing insights and special moments
A post-reflection, however,
definitely is not a post-game analysis
of *whys* and *should-haves*

For simplicity
the following instructions
usually use female gender pronouns
Modify as necessary

Most of all,
Enjoy!

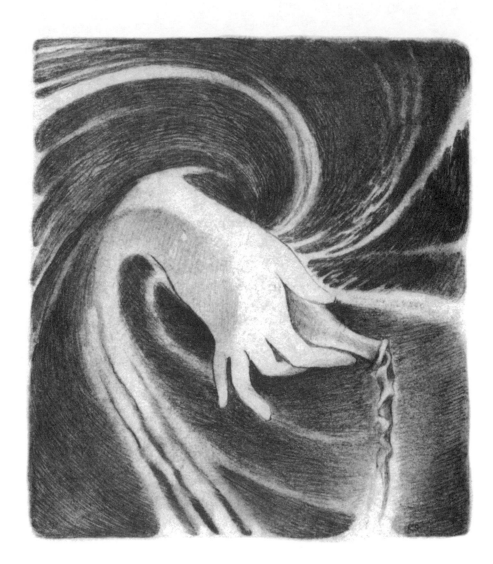

3 Ritual Accouterments
Accessories

MUSIC

The most conducive music
       for most sensual ceremonies
          is without lyrics
          and usually without dominating rhythms
    Words encourage thinking
       which often is a distraction
          from sensation and feeling experiences
  And when the rhythm is obvious
       we might follow the music's beat
       rather than the receiver's

There is an increasing selection
       of audio cassettes / compact disks
       for calming and nourishing the body/mind
Possibilities include environmental recordings and
       meditational music
While many classical selections
       are very beautiful,
    the moods, dynamics, and rhythms
       frequently have a predominating influence
Experimentation is the key

OILS, LOTIONS, SOAPS

A good choice for massage oil
        is a pure, unscented vegetable oil
    Coconut oil is excellent
        though it solidifies
            at less-than-warm temperatures
    Other possibilities are
        plain almond oil, apricot kernel oil, and safflower oil
            all of which can be purchased at
                natural food stores and maybe supermarkets

You can add fragrances
        to these oils
        but not too much
    Sometimes fragrance ingredients are irritating
        to the skin and especially membranous tissues
    Some consider mineral oil
            to be unhealthy on or in our bodies
        Its advantage is
            it does not leave a rancid smell in sheets
        Baby oil is simply mineral oil with fragrance added

Most lotions have a number of additives
        and they usually evaporate or soak in
            before you finish massaging
    However, when mixed with oil
        they create a wonderfully sensual texture
            for hand and feet massage

Among soaps
        the liquid variety may be easier to use
    Usually they can be purchased at natural food stores
    Some find peppermint liquid soap especially pleasing
        but may be a little too mentholated
        for the genital/anal areas

Unfortunately many of the commercial *love oils* and *love lotions*
        leave much to be desired
    especially if you were to ingest them
Use caution
    if the ingredients are not listed
        or if the listed ingredients are unfamiliar
            or include additives or preservatives

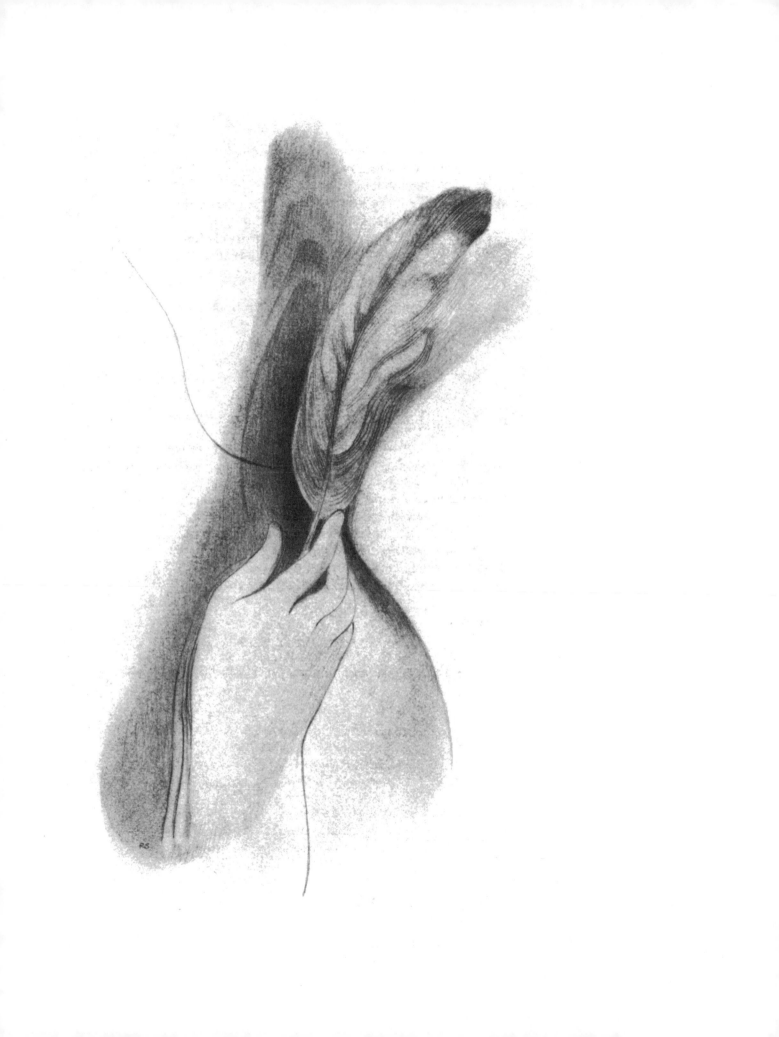

BATHING ACCESSORIES

A natural sponge and a loofa mitt
        are favorites in the bath
    Synthetic sponges may not feel aesthetically pleasing
    When the loofa is of a mitt variety
           (one side of loofa, the other side of cloth)
        you can put one on each hand
    These are often available at natural food stores
        bath boutiques, and some cosmetic shops

Air pillow head rests for the bath
    are great and are obtainable at bath boutiques

Hydrojets, either from portable or installed units
        are fun but may be overpowering
        in a nurturing ceremony

Rinsing with a hand-held container
    —the rhythm
        of pouring and then dipping for more water—
           creates a calming trance
    Since glass can break
         and metal can be cumbersome and noisy
        select a plastic container
           perhaps about ten inches long
           and four inches wide
    Shower attachments that vary the water flow
        are an alternative

FEATHERS AND FAVORITE FABRICS

Ostrich and peacock plumage
        are especially pleasurable
    Peacock feathers may be available
        at shops that carry dried flowers,
           while ostrich feathers may be difficult to find

Silky and furry fabrics
    are other favorites

MASSAGE TABLES

When giving a massage,
       for most, a massage table
             is best
Alternatively
          place a foam pad and sheet
               on a sturdy dining room table
               or a banquet table
                    (the kind with folding legs)

You may find other accouterments pleasing to the senses
       browsing in shops specializing in oils and soaps
            in bath shops
            and in sensuous boutiques especially for lovers
Still,
       your attentive presence
            with your beloved
       is the most important gift

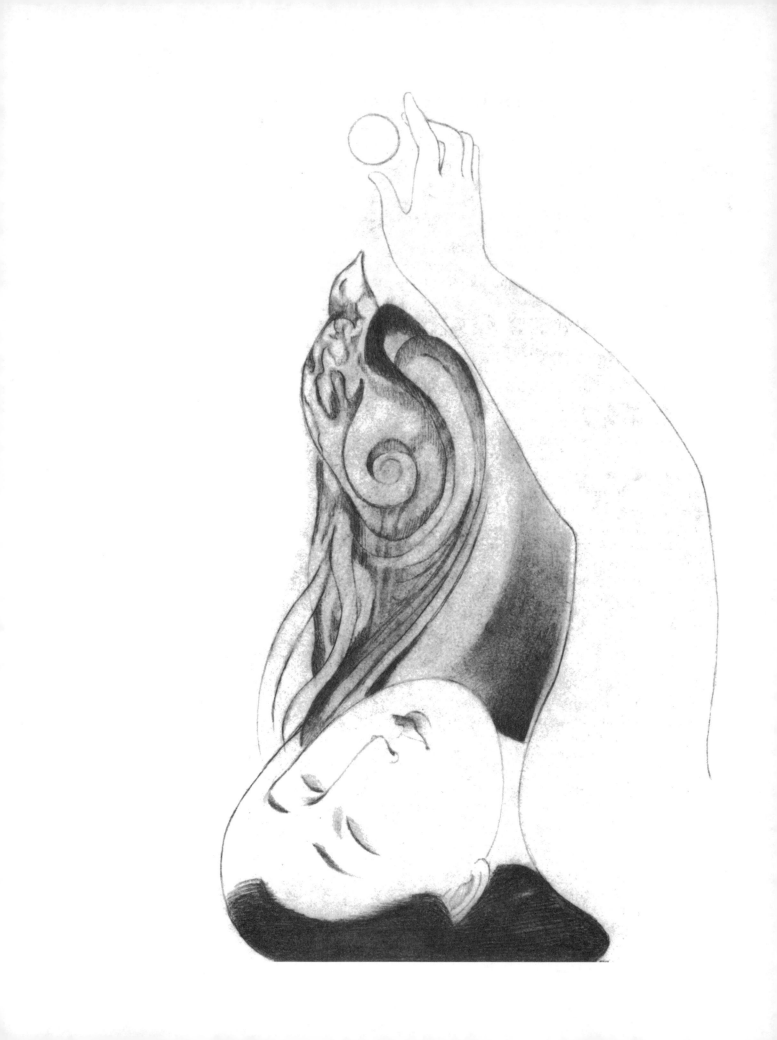

4 The Inner Garden
Guided Imagery

Lie back
Let go
Begin to hear the waves
Feel the soft sand beneath you
> *the sun's rays above you*
>> *bathing each cell in warmth*
> *the sea breezes caressing your skin*
Let go . . .

The adventures of the mind
> are immense
> We can journey into richness and depth
>> beyond time and location
> To enter into this adventure,
>> we allow
>>> logic, reason, and comparison
>> to be neither guide nor excess baggage

In ceremony
> we are able
>> to touch a deeper inner peace
> Here we can expand
>> our intuitive awareness
> Sensation and feeling
>> become alive
> We taste a forgotten nectar

As the giver
> you become a guide
Your words
>> soft in tone
>> slow in pace
> lead your beloved into sanctuary

GUIDELINES

When you communicate instructions
> or lead a guided imagery
>> be nondemanding
> Never express judgment, anger, or impatience
>> through voice or actions
> Laughter as a shared joy, however, is a delight
Let your voice
> be soft and gentle
>> almost as if lullabying an infant

To begin
> invite the recipient
>> to remove her shoes
>> and to loosen tight clothing
> Alternatively
>> she might be in a robe or nude
> Contact lenses may require removal

Next assist her to sit or lie down comfortably
> Be certain that she feels warm
>> as the body generates little heat
>> in a guided imagery

Now suggest that she close her eyes
> and bring her awareness
> to her breath
>> taking a few fuller inhalations
> Perhaps give a laying on of hands
>> on her abdomen and forehead

After about five minutes of these relaxation inductions
> she will likely be ready
>> for an inner journey

Your *imagery introduction* might be like this:

> Now I am going to invite you to imagine an event.
> Whatever comes into your awareness is perfect,
> even if it does not fit my words. There are no right or
> wrong experiences. Allow whatever comes up to
> come up. While I may say "imagine" or "visualize,"
> be open to feeling, sensing, intuiting, and any other
> means of perception available to you. If you are not
> aware of a response, allow that to be OK. Be open to
> experiencing any feeling or sensation in your body.

Now explore the following inner journey
      (Perhaps make the guided imagery
         a ceremony in itself)
  Present the wording
      as your own creation
      rather than simply reading it
(A "..." means to take a longer pause
      perhaps about ten seconds)
There is no need to be dramatic
      Yet, allow feeling in the delivery

The recipient
      may become very deeply relaxed
She may even appear to be asleep
      Do not worry
      Most likely she is soaring
Simply continue guiding the imagery
      If she should be asleep
         know that she is receiving a needed rest

THE EARTH COMMUNION IMAGERY

Here we give thanks
      to the beauty and nourishment
         our planet provides
Begin with the relaxation inductions and imagery introduction
      Perhaps be aware
         of your own inner images as you speak

> I'd like you to begin to imagine yourself walking
> down a path in a forest. Let it be an imaginary for-
> est. It is a beautiful and serene place...

Now begin to be aware of how your feet feel as you walk down the path. You may have on boots or shoes. Perhaps you are wearing sandals, or maybe you're barefoot. Feel the texture, the softness or the hardness of the earth each time your foot touches the ground. Notice if the path is narrow or wide. Notice if it is rocky or maybe muddy. Hear the sound of your footsteps. Let this be very real for you. Whatever feelings you have are fine. This forest is a special place. There is a richness and a beauty here. Allow your senses to perceive and to enjoy...

As you walk down this path begin to notice the trees around you. As the sunlight comes through the trees, see the shadows. Also, notice the subtle changes in the forest colors. Look all around you and perceive all the varying shapes...

Smell all the wonderful fragrances that the breezes bring. There are some places where the sun is more intense and you can smell the warmth. The places in the shade may have a different fragrance. There's a world of many subtle smells along this path. Allow yourself to experience them...

From time to time you may hear birds sing and other sounds of the forest. Maybe you can hear the trees creaking as the winds swish through their branches. You might even hear small animals scurrying through the brush...

Be open to feeling peaceful on this path. Allow yourself to be with each step, each vision, each fragrance. To commune with nature is precious. Allow yourself this...

Walking down the path, you'll find there is a clearing off to the side, maybe like a meadow, where it is soft and very easy to rest. When you see this clearing, walk over to it. As you enter, you can even smell the warmth of the sun. Find a comfortable place to lie down there. Notice how easy it is to totally let go and to allow all your muscles to relax. Feel yourself being supported by the earth beneath you. There is nothing to do except to let go...

As you rest there, begin to become aware of the warmth of the sun that comes to touch your skin. Even through your clothing you can feel the warmth. The rays penetrate each cell of your body. You can feel a gentle tingling as the cells are bathed in the sun's energy. Feel it penetrating all the way to the core of your body, nurturing you. Allow yourself to melt into the earth...

Let's take a moment to give thanks. To give thanks to life. To give thanks to the beauty of Earth. To give thanks to the warmth of the sun. To give thanks to the breezes and the fragrances they bring. To give thanks for the abundance of food. To give thanks for the water. This is a special place where we live. All we have to do is to open ourselves to perceive and enjoy these abundant gifts. With your inner voice take a moment to give thanks to this planet...

OK. Let's begin to come back now. Know that these images and feelings are available to you anytime you wish. Begin to take some fuller breaths. Perhaps inhale and hold your breath a couple of seconds before letting go... Begin to feel your body as it rests here on the bed (carpet, etc.). Come back even more. And when you feel ready, open your eyes and share your experiences with me.

(If this guided imagery is the beginning of a longer ceremony, perhaps the verbal sharing would be better after the whole ceremony.)

When she returns
    be present
    be close

This is one of many possible inner journeys
    Create your own if you wish
        Use memories or make-believe
        Visit the future
        Visit the past
            different cultures
            different lifetimes
    Explore one of these scenes:
        sitting on a secluded beach
        listening to a babbling brook
        drifting on a raft down a lazy river
        soaring on the back of a large silver-white bird

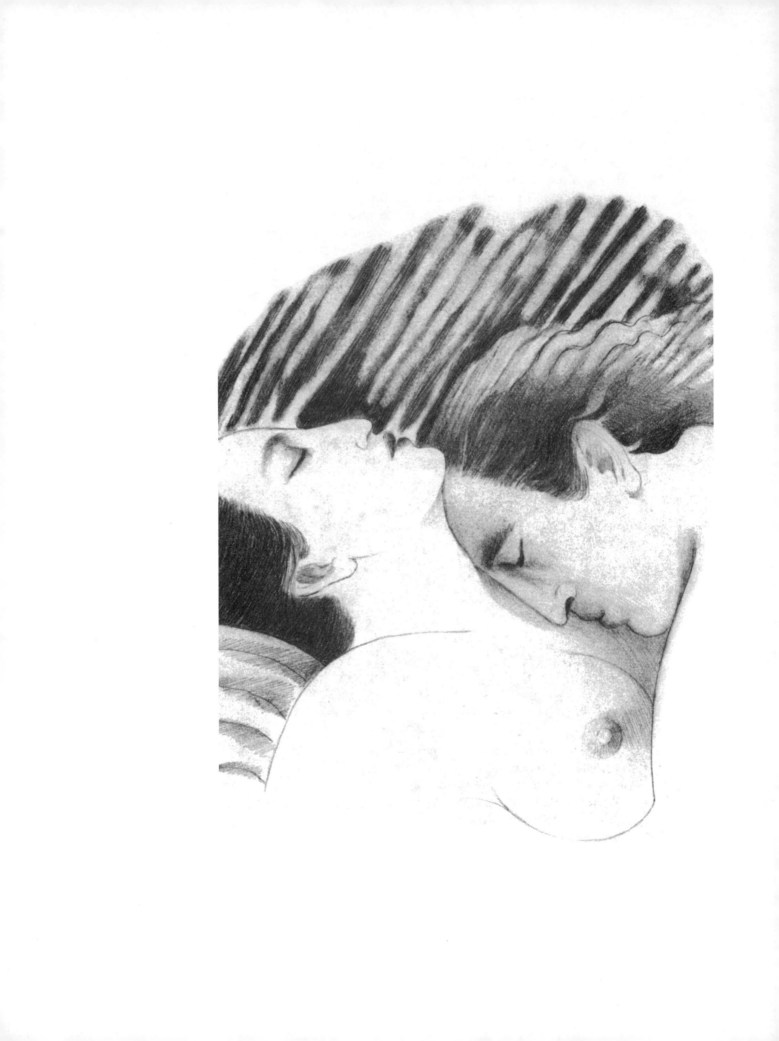

5 Sensual Communion
Feeding

Smell
Taste
Savor
Slow down
> _Feel_
> _Let the moment last_
Linger in the energy

WHAT TO FEED

Is there food or drink
> the recipient dislikes or excludes from her diet?
Any allergies?
> Ask her if you do not know
> Ask a friend if you wish to surprise
Perhaps serve the following suggestions
> Perhaps be adventurous

Sparkling Nectars or Other Beverages

Sparkling apple cider or sparkling grape juice
> often are first choices
Usually one bottle is sufficient
Fruit juices, especially very cold apple juice,

or a multiple-fruit purée
titillate tastes as well
If you prefer champagne
select a very dry or brut variety
Wine is probably better accompanying meals

Fruits

These are some favorites
mangoes, papayas, kiwis
strawberries, bananas
apples (a sweet variety such as Red or Golden Delicious)
persimmons, fresh berries
grapes (preferably seedless)
watermelon, nectarines, peaches
plums, cherries
Other possibilities are
pears, cantaloupes and other melons
coconuts, pomegranates
oranges, grapefruits, pineapples
Though be cautious
mixing citrus or other acid-tasting fruits
with whipped cream and nuts
Usually you need purchase only
one piece of each fruit
except for the berries, grapes, and strawberries
Variety is the key
There are seasonal variations and
markets vary in quality

Nuts

Nuts provide a crunchy, chewy contrast
to fruit and whipped cream
Perhaps serve a single variety of nut
that enhances rather than dominates other flavors
Almonds are an excellent choice
Other selections might be walnuts or pecans

Whipped Cream

The texture and the taste of whipped cream
either hand-whipped or electric-beater-whipped
can be incredible

WHAT
To
FEED

A half pint or pint of the thickest cream is plenty
      Save *prewhipped* whipped cream for a last resort
      Use whipped cream substitutes
            only when dietary restrictions necessitate

Alternatively, prepare a fruit sauce
      of honey or maple syrup
            with a half or whole pint of plain sour cream
            or plain yogurt

Other Possibilities

The following
      are not likely to be favorites
      but you can explore them

In general, a mild cheese
      is more likely to blend
      than a sharp variety
      Fruit-flavored cheeses are often very interesting
Do not overdo the cheese and crackers
      — a heavy stomach in a sensual ceremony
          would be a distraction

Candies,
      such as extra fine chocolate,
and baked desserts
      might be all right
but only in very small amounts
      and only when especially desired
Candies have a tendency
      to overwhelm the taste buds
and baked desserts may be too filling

Given an emphasis on fruit,
      hors d'oeuvres or any salty or tart delight
         might clash
When uncertain
      try them yourself before the ceremony

Some tantric sexual rituals
      use grains and meats
You can experiment with these
      after becoming familiar with the preceding suggestions

Sensual Ceremony

153

PREPARATION AND ARRANGEMENT

To have fully ripened fruit
        you may need to shop a few days before your ceremony
Canned, frozen, or unnecessarily processed ingredients
        are only as a last resort

To prepare and arrange the ceremonial platter
        anticipate at least an hour
While the recipient will see the design
        on the ceremonial platter for a few minutes only,
        her memory may last for a lifetime

You may need the following
- a platter: a little larger than a standard dining plate
    perhaps of clear glass or stainless steel
- a cutting board and a knife for the fruit
- a serving spoon
- utensils for preparing the whipped cream or sauce
- one or two champagne glasses
    perhaps a tulip shaped wine glass
      rather than the standard champagne glass

For the first step
    make the sparkling nectar
      (a sparkling cider/juice or champagne)
    very cold
If the ceremony location is a hotel or motel
    have the beverage very cold before leaving home
      since some ice buckets have only a chilling effect
If possible, chill the glasses

Next prepare the whipped cream
    Hand whisking requires extensive energy
      but the texture is sometimes finer
      than that from an electric beater
The whipping is often easier
    if the mixing bowl and whipping cream are cold
During the whipping
    add about two teaspoons of sugar
      and perhaps a little vanilla
    Real maple syrup is another possible sweetener
      added according to taste
      though some find the flavor too strong
Be careful not to whip too long
    as you might produce butter
If you are going to take the whipped cream to another location
    you can put it in a plastic container with a lid

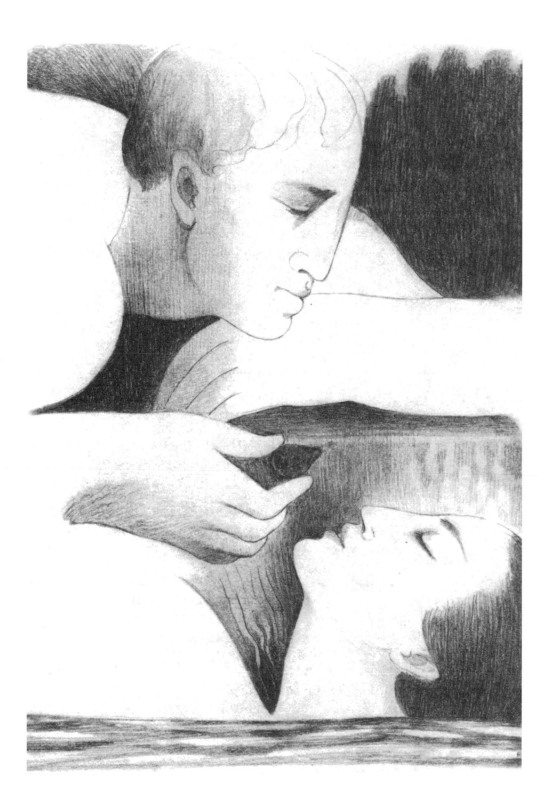

To prepare a fruit sauce
      of honey or maple syrup with sour cream or yogurt,
   heat the honey or maple syrup
      until it almost begins to simmer
   Then pour and mix it
      into the sour cream or yogurt
      Continue tasting until lightly sweetened

Some suggestions for preparing the fruits
   First, wash thoroughly
      and taste each fruit for texture and ripeness
   Purchasing a wide variety of fruits
      ensures quality

- kiwi
      cut off the ends, and quarter lengthwise, with skin on
- papaya
      cut in half lengthwise and scoop out all the seeds
- mango
      cut lengthwise along each side of the large seed
        On each of the two serving sections
         make horizontal and vertical slices
          (in the meat, not the skin)
        and then curl the section inside out
- persimmon
      slice the skin from the tipped point
        (like petals of a flower)
      and gently fold back the slices
- grapes
      leave clustered on the branch
- strawberries
      perhaps leave the stems on until serving
- apple and pear
      quarter and slice vertically into thin slices
      Slice just before presenting
        or sprinkle lime or lemon juice on the slices
- banana
      slice into small cross sections

The arrangement
      depends on which fresh fruits are available
      as well as the size and shape of the serving platter
   Here are some possibilities
      Line the banana slices
        on the outer rim of the platter
      Then on each slice
        place a single almond
          systematically pointing in some direction
      Apple slices could also line the outer rim

Fill the papaya with whipped cream
     and a strawberry or cherry on top
     A champagne glass is an alternative to the papaya
Use the different colors of the fruits in the design

Never let the recipient see the preparation process
   Upon completion
     cover and hide the platter
     so that she does not have a sneak preview
       and the cat does not get into the whipped cream
   Keeping the preparation in the refrigerator, though,
     may over-chill the fruit

A few extra pointers
     when the ceremony is given in a hotel or motel room
   Order ice and an ice bucket
     a good while before the ceremony
   In most hotels you can also order
      a spoon, glasses, and a platter or large plate
     A good cutting knife may not be available to guests
     If room service hesitates about delivering
       without a food or drink purchase,
     offer to pay for the usage
One final touch,
     if you are using a tray, you can also place on it
     a small vase with a single flower

FEEDING CEREMONIES

While you are making the final touches
     the recipient can be relaxing
     listening to quiet music
   Or she could be by the fireplace
     sipping hot tea
Hearing the nearby sounds of food preparation
     may build suspense
      if she can not see the activity
Soften the lights if possible
Unplug the telephone
     eliminate other possible interruptions
And do not burn incense
     too soon before the actual feeding

A feeding ceremony
     can be in combination with a bathing
      as in a Secret Garden Ceremony

or it can be a ceremony in itself
Here are some guidelines
common to both situations

Present the platter for a visual feast
Let it say
"This is just for you"
Then ask if there is anything there
that she wishes not to eat
After setting the platter down
ask if she would like
to be surprised
or to request
If "to be surprised" is the response
invite her to close her eyes
If the mood shifts to requesting
flow with it
When feeding
slowly place the selection just in front of her lips
so that she can smell the aromas
If she is not aware of the presence
very lightly touch the food to her lips
This feeding is not intended
as a guessing game about what is served
Now is a time for her to be in the direct experience
of taste and smell
rather than discussing the topic
Gently encourage focusing on the sensations
Feed with your fingers
An inch above her tongue
squeeze grapes, strawberries, or watermelon
and let the sweet juices drop
drip by drip
When serving
vary the flavors and textures
Explore combinations
Feed slowly
Wait until she has thoroughly savored
the previous serving
If you should wish to taste also
first ask permission to serve yourself
Should she want to feed you
remind her that this is a time
for her to be served
She can give that as a gift another time
Exceptions are always negotiable
At some point let her know that she is to indicate
when she is satiated

THE EPICUREAN BATH

This is a very special, unique gift
    It is simply the combination
        of feeding and bathing in a bath
    Certain exquisite experiences
        are far more accessible *in* a bath
            than outside of a bath
    Before giving an epicurean bath
        become familiar with the ceremonial bathing
            in the next chapter

After you escort the recipient to the bath
    perhaps leave momentarily
        to give her an opportunity
        to adjust to the womb-like environment
    When you return
        you can be nude
            carrying the platter of delights,
            the sparkling nectar, a glass, and a spoon
    Immediately but without rushing
        present the platter for her visual feast

Serve the sparkling nectar or other beverage first
    If it is champagne
        place a cloth over the cork
        and pointing it away from her and yourself
            slowly twist or rock the cork back and forth
            until it gently pops
    Pour the sparkling nectar into the glass
        Without rushing
            place the sparkling bubbles under her nose
            to be inhaled
    If she reaches up as if to serve herself
        remove the glass to say nonverbally
            "Please allow yourself to be served"
    Usually by the second or third removal
        your communication is clear

Cup Runneth Over

After a while
    there is a special way
        to serve a sparkling nectar
    Perhaps warn the recipient by asking
        "Are you ready for something delightfully different?"
    As she is sipping

allow the sparkling nectar
to run over onto her chin and chest
Her first response may be
shock at the temperature
If she is appalled by the *waste*
this is the perfect time
to lavish even more upon her body
Also be sensitive to the possibility
that she may find the sensations undesirable
and be prepared to stop

Sparkling Shower

If she especially enjoys the sparkling thrills above
invite her to stand
Step into the tub and embrace her
Then pour directly from the bottle
so that the bubbles slither down
between your chests, abdomens, and pelvises
Hopefully there is something to lean against
—it may be difficult to stand up at this point
After a while invite her to resume sitting
and continue the feeding

Sparkling Kiss

Take a sip of sparkling nectar
and while kissing her
allow it to flow from your lips

Sparkling Massage

Take a large sip of sparkling nectar without swallowing
Then place your mouth
on her neck, breasts, fingers, toes, or elsewhere
and give an oral massage
as the sparkling essence seeps through your lips

Palm Sundae

An advantage to feeding in the bath
is that if anything slips from your hands or her lips
the experience can be a part of the ceremony

Place whipped cream and several fruits
  such as banana, mango, papaya, and strawberries
    in your palm
With the edge of the spoon
  make a sort of purée
Next, place your closed palm against her lips
Squeeze
  and slowly ooze the lusciousness
    through her lips

Creaming and Papaya Pleasure

Wait until she feels sufficiently fed
  before beginning these next treats
  She may be uninterested in eating more afterward
For Creaming
  abundantly stroke whipped cream
    over her chest, abdomen, arms, and legs
  She may wish then
    that you taste your creamed creation
Creaming with the sour cream and honey sauce
  is too sticky for most people
Here as always
  avoid sugared ingredients in the vaginal area
    as this might lead to yeast difficulties

Follow with Papaya Pleasure
  or Persimmon Pleasure, or Mango Pleasure
As with the cream
  slide the fruit all over her body
With the persimmon
  first remove the seed if necessary
With the papaya and mango
  shape the fruit so that the soft, fleshy meat
    comes fully in contact with her skin
Sometimes in Creaming or Papaya Pleasure
  the recipient goes into a partial trance
  Do not worry
Following this
  pour water on her for several minutes
Now bathe with soap and water
  as described in the next chapter

FEEDING OUTSIDE THE BATH

There are other locations for a feeding ceremony,
        the floor, the bed, or any comfortable place in nature
    Here the recipient's position
        is lying down on her back
    This body position and nonbath setting
        usually create a quite different mood
            than in the Epicurean Bath

Invite the recipient to lie down
    with her head in your lap
    She can lie so that you face her feet
        or she can be perpendicular to you
    Perhaps place a pillow under her head
        as well as underneath yourself
    This position necessitates chewing
        rather than gulping the food
    However, since drinking
        is very difficult in this position
            provide plenty of juicy fruit
        (A possible option
            would be to provide a straw that bends
            or a wine-carrying pouch with a spout)

Between each feeding
    stroke her hair and brow
        These caresses help relax her even more
    In general, the greater the relaxation
        the more pleasurable the tastes
    From time to time
        use a napkin or damp cloth
            to very gently wipe off excesses
            from her chin and cheeks
    When she is full
        continue stroking for a while
            perhaps with a facial massage

At the end of the ceremony
    she may feel very relaxed and nurtured

Rest

Cuddle

Feel

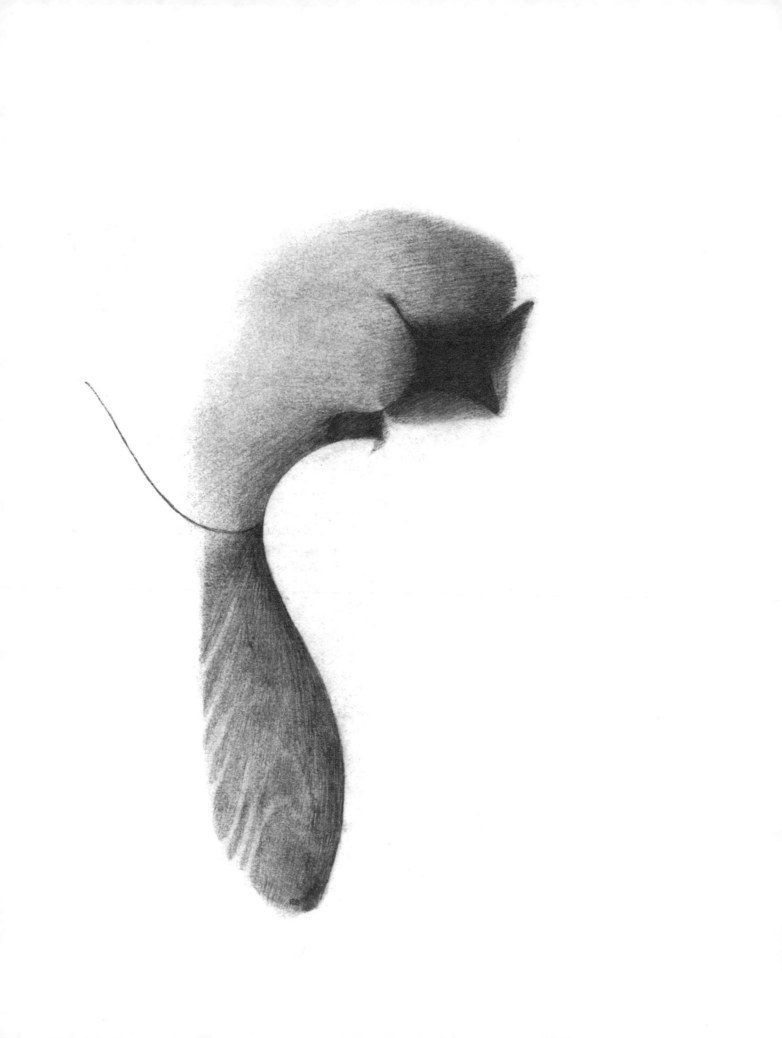

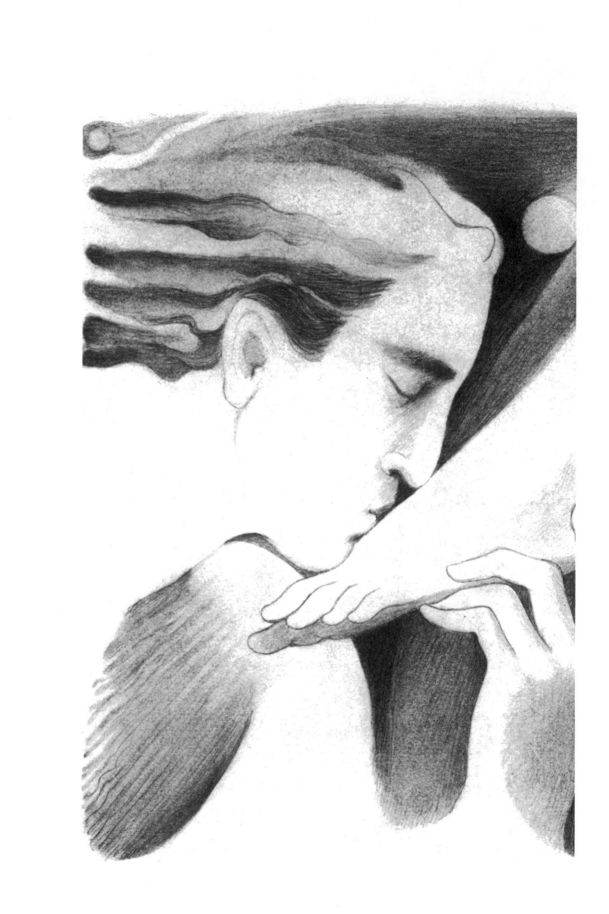

6 Ceremonial Waters
Body and Foot Bathing

Soft
Warm
Soothing
Boundless
Enter into the ceremonial waters

A pool or stream in nature
             a bathtub
             a basin
             a shower
             a hot tub
     Ceremonial waters abound

In a Secret Garden Ceremony
             a bathtub is usually the location of choice
     There is privacy and no insect intrusions
             the recipient can recline
             the water temperature is easily adjustable

For a shorter ceremony
         a foot bathing is especially nurturing
             Also, it can be easily given
                 to someone who is not a sexual partner

BODY BATHING

If you are giving a bathtub bath,
  a home or hotel/motel
  are the most likely environments
 At home you have many comforts
   but may need to make extensive rearrangements
    to the ceremonial bathing area
 When making a reservation at a hotel or motel
   confirm that the bath is not only a shower stall

Accessories

There are several essentials
  hot water
  soap
  towels
  and something for pouring water

Liquid soap with peppermint or almond essence
  are many people's preference
   Purchase them at health food or natural food stores

Select a towel to cover a cold tile floor
   if the bath mat is missing
  You may need a washcloth for cooling the recipient's brow
  For drying
   reserve at least three bath towels
  And if you are including feeding
   a small towel may be necessary for your hands
  In most hotels you will have to order additional towels

For pouring water
   use either a container, or a natural sponge, or both
  An ideal pouring container in a bathtub
   is plastic
   and about a foot long and four inches in diameter
  Larger or bulky containers
   may make water dipping very difficult
  And glass containers are elegant but breakable

Other nice accessories are
   a candle, loofas, a bath brush
   fragrances for the bath water
   maybe bubble bath or bath salt ingredients

a bath pillow, possibly a rubber stopper
plants, and music

A candle is almost a necessity
Its flame transforms
Place the candle
either at the foot of the tub
or in front of a mirror

Loofas are the thick fibrous interiors of a type of fruit
When they are wet
they create an exciting sensation on the skin
especially on the bottom of the feet
the buttocks, and the back
With a loofa mitt
(a loofa on one side
and a washcloth on the other)
you can have one on each hand

Natural-fiber bath brushes create an exotic sensation
similar to the loofa

Delicate fragrances arising from the bath
deepen the involvement of the senses
The fragrances might come from bath salts,
bath oils, or bubble bath added to the water
Prior to putting anything in the bath water
ask if the future recipient's skin is sensitive
to any ingredients
Also, be cautious of synthetic chemical scents and colors
that are in many products

One method of adding fragrances is
to put one or two drops (careful, not too much)
of essential oil of lemon, orange, spearmint,
or peppermint
into the stream of hot water
when the bath is almost full
Another way is to steep herbs enclosed in a cloth bag
as you begin drawing the bath

A bath pillow, purchased from a bath shop
comforts the recipient's neck and head
Rolled-up towels are a substitute
but have a tendency to slide into the water

Occasionally a bath drain plug
will not make a complete seal

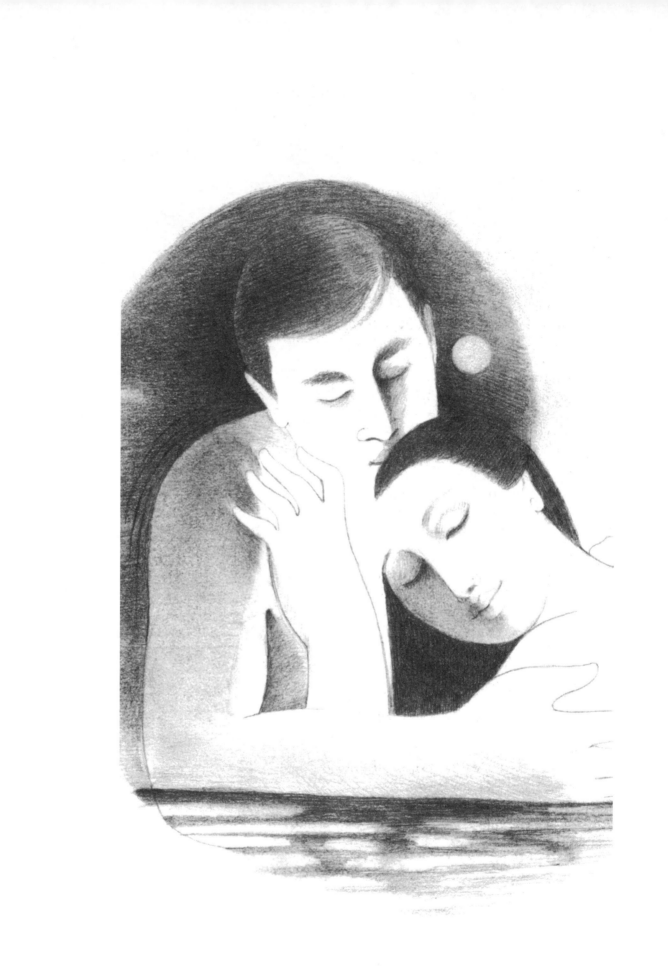

Before using an unfamiliar tub
    perhaps purchase a flat rubber disk
    at a hardware store

Plants, if easily available, add ambiance

In a ceremonial bath
    music with candle light creates an encompassing dome
      separating you and your special friend
      from the outside world
    The selection of music, however, is a crucial step
      to be taken before the day of the bath
    Disco and rap music will probably not be in harmony
      with the mood
    In most cases
      a portable cassette tape player is quite suitable

And if you wish
    a rubber ducky

Preparations

These are the behind-the-scenes preparations
    to eliminate potential distractions
    and to add to the nuances

In a massage
    the recipient's eyes are closed
  In a bath
    her eyes are often open
Here are some ways to nurture the visual sense as well

Remove the shower curtain
    and if possible, the shower curtain bar
  The sliding bath doors, however,
      might be a real stumbling block
    You may need a regular or Phillips screwdriver
    With perseverance, ingenuity,
      and sometimes brute force
    most sliding doors will come off
  If they just won't come off,
    adapt the ceremony
      by sliding the doors back and forth as needed
    (You will want to place a rolled towel
      between your buttocks and the metal tracks
        on which the doors slide)

If the tub itself does not appear or feel clean
    bathe it
Be sure to rinse off all of the cleanser
      — sandpaper is no fun
Even clean out the soap dish
    and the upper corners of the tub

Next remove almost everything that is movable
    in the bathing room
Start with the shampoo bottle
    all the bars of soap
    the toothpaste tops
    the shaving utensils
    the toilet brush
    the wastepaper basket
      almost everything
Remove reading materials from sight
Any towels not intended to be used
    can be placed elsewhere
(Exceptions might be a decorative object
    and the roll of toilet paper on the holder)

Most important,
    remember everything's original location
    as well as where you hide it
    After the ceremony
      you will put everything back in place

Here are some additions

Perhaps minimize outside light
    If there are windows or a skylight
      you might cover them with a towel or dark sheet
    Though when the window is large and the view is beautiful
      it may be best to leave it uncovered

Now the water
    If you are not sure how much hot water is available
      run a half tub of hot water
        about a half hour before the beginning of the bath
      Then just prior to the beginning
        more hot water will likely be available
    Test the water temperature with your foot or inner forearm
    Be sure to check it again
      just before inviting your guest into the bathing room
    When the bath is almost full
      is the best time to add fragrances, bath oils
        or bubble bath
      Herbs can be added at the beginning
        since they usually need to steep

One more suggestion,
      if the toilet is in the same room as the bath
            use it before escorting in the recipient
      There may not be an opportune moment
            during the one- to two-hour ceremony

Now you are ready
      for your guest of honor

THE BATHING CEREMONY

Beginning

Candle lit
      water temperature tested
            music on?

If you have a kimono
      wear it to greet the recipient
            who is in another room relaxing, possibly in a robe

Bow and announce to her
            "Your bath is prepared"
      Then escort her into the bathing room

Now you can either undress her
      or invite her to disrobe
            and sit in the bath while you momentarily leave
      But before leaving
            inform her how to adjust the hot and cold water
                just in case
      Leaving the room for a few minutes
            allows her to use the toilet
            and then settle into the warm bath water
                the fragrances, and the candle light
      You can disrobe before returning

Almost anything we do with soap and water
            can easily create a ceremonial feeling
      When you are ready to bathe
            try the following sequence
      Bathing is relatively free-form
      However, you can use massage strokes as guidelines

Remember to have fun
 Getting her clean
  is not the objective here

Feet and Legs

Begin with your feet in the water
  and sitting on the tub rim near the recipient's feet
 Gracefully lift one of her legs
  to rest on your thigh,
   the one nearest the foot end of the tub
 After applying soap to your hands
  spread it on the foot and leg
 Use soap abundantly
  Move slowly, attentively
 After using varying movements and pressures
  for several minutes,
  stroke the bottom of the foot with a loofa
   if one is available
  (Make sure the loofa has softened
   by soaking it a few seconds first)
 Perhaps using a sponge
  now pour water over her leg and foot
 There is no need, however,
  to restrict the pouring to just the soapy areas

When the first leg is completed
 gently lower it back into the bath
  and raise the other leg onto your thigh
 Repeat the lathering, stroking, and water pouring

Arms and Hands

Slide up the tub rim to reach the arms

A hint,
 if the receiver is shorter than the bathtub
  there is a tendency
   for her to slide down towards the foot end
 The solution is to place your foot
  (the one nearest the foot end of the tub)
  between her legs
  so that her pelvic floor rests against your ankle
 This gentle pressure on the pelvis often feels comforting

Once established
    lather, stroke, and rinse one arm and hand
       and then the other
    For some, a loofa is too rough here

Front Torso

Now bathe the abdomen, chest, and breast areas
    For the portion of the body underneath water
       apply even more soap

On the abdomen
      make circular movements
    This is also a good position
      from which to bathe the pelvic area
    Be careful using peppermint soap
      if you include
      the vaginal or anal membranous tissue areas
        —the mentholated effect might be too much

If the bath water has cooled
      add more hot water
        evenly distributing it by stirring
    With the chest exposed to the cooler air
      it is particularly nice to pour water there
    The warmth and soft flow on the heart
      are very nurturing

Hair Washing

If the recipient wishes
    you can wash her hair
      either before or after washing her back
    However, it seems in most situations
      the hair washing is best given as a ceremony
      in itself
    After an extensive bath
      the mood is usually more conducive
      to lying down, resting, perhaps cuddling
      than drying and brushing
        Experiment for yourself
    Whenever you give a hair washing
      use plenty of lather
    And when pouring water
      check with her regarding the water temperature

If the hair is washed during a body bath
remember to rinse with fresh water

Back

Sitting in the tub to give the back bathing
is wonderfully cozy
If it is desirable and possible to get into the tub
invite her to sit up slowly
and slide forward a few feet
Then cuddle in from behind
with your legs spread to each side
While she is leaning forward
with her head relaxed downward
lather up the back

Extra attention
to the upper back and shoulders
is special
Sliding your thumbs down along the grooves
just to each side of the spine is likewise

Two loofa mitts can double the pleasure
Be firm sliding them downward on each side of the spine
though too many passes can be irritating

Now with the container
pour water over the back
for a minute or two

Conclusion of Bathing

Invite her to lean back slowly
onto your chest
Continue pouring the water
for several more minutes
Pouring from this position
can be a little awkward
but it is worth it
Remember, there is no rush

Once you've completed the pouring
simply hold her
perhaps with one of your hands resting on her abdomen
and the other hand over her heart

Then most importantly
        follow her breath
           and breathe in unison:
    Inhale as she inhales
       exhale as she exhales

Breathe like this for maybe five or ten minutes
    Perhaps by then
       time will have disappeared

Drying Off

When it comes time to leave the bath
      ask her to lean forward
      and remain there while you get up
        and prepare for the drying

Once you are ready
      suggest that she rise S L O W L Y
    Assist with your hands
      — it may not be easy to stand up
      and step out of a tub after a bath like this

Now begin the drying
    On the upper part of the body
      wrap one towel from the back
      and one from the front
    If her hair is wet
      take a separate towel to dry it a little
    Next, with a combination
      of patting
      and sliding your hands up and down and in circles
        over the towel surface,
      dry her back, front torso, and arms
    If the towels do not reach down to her hands
      use a separate towel

Leaving the towels on the upper portion of the body
      dry one leg at a time
      with the up and down and circular motions
        over the towel surface
    Make sure the inner thighs, genitals, and inner buttocks
      are dried
    With a fresh towel
      gently pat dry her face and neck

Ask if anywhere still feels damp

Next ask if she wishes to lie down
    On a bed or in front of a fireplace
        may be options
    If you are planning to give a massage
        direct her to the massage location

To assist in the transition
        out of this etheric bathing womb,
    inform her before opening the door
        that outside
            the light may be brighter
                and the air cooler

If you wish
    you can present
        the rubber ducky as a memento afterward

FOOT BATHING CEREMONY

If you want to give a gift
    that is both relaxing and simple
        a foot bathing is perfect
Of all the techniques presented in this book
    the foot bathing
        is the most widely applicable
        to friends who are not sexual partners
Grandparents, bosses, employees, teachers
        and many others
        can be profoundly nurtured

What You Need

These are the basics
    which may already be around the house
    soap, perhaps liquid soap
    a plastic basin
        or any container large enough for at least one foot
    at least three towels

Additionally there could be
    a large, comfortable chair for the recipient
    relaxing music in the background
    and elimination of possible disruptions
        such as the telephone

As the giver
>you may want to sit on a pillow or cushion
>to lessen any strain on your legs and hips

Initial Steps

Perhaps lower the lights
>put on soothing music
>light a candle
>and do anything else to create a desirable ambiance

Then with your friend relaxing in a comfortable chair
>>lying on the carpet
>>or lying on a bed with her knees bending over the edge
>draw the water in the basin
>Usually the temperature is best
>>very warm bordering on hot
>You can always add hot water later
>>after her feet have become accustomed to the heat
>If, however, the weather outside is really hot
>>lukewarm or cool water may be preferable

Take off her shoes and socks
>Since most people are not used
>>>to having this done for them
>>you may have to use gentle, verbal persuasion
>If there are stockings
>>she may have to remove them
>Next you roll up pants legs or skirts
>>to about the knee

This is also a good time
>to invite your friend to allow the eyes to close
>>first removing contact lenses if necessary

After placing a towel underneath her feet
>slide the basin near them
>Lift one of her legs
>>supporting it
>>>at the bottom of the foot
>>>and at the calf or underneath the knee
>>Actually what you are doing
>>>is nonverbally communicating to her
>>>to let go and to allow herself to be taken care of
>Place your lower hand
>>so that it will enter the water first
>>in case the temperature is too hot

If there is space
        place the second foot in the basin also

Important,
        make sure that her toes are not jammed
                into the end of the basin
        and that the rim of the basin is not wedged into her calves

Sometimes it's nice to let your friend rest in solitude
        with her feet soaking for a short while

Bathing The Feet

Begin the bathing
        with a laying on of hands in the water
    One hand is on the side of the foot
        the other is on top
    Close your eyes
        and let your hands relax into the touch
                and the warmth of the water

After a minute or so
        lift the foot and leg
        and bring it out of the water
                to rest on the towel or your leg
    With a little maneuvering
        slide the basin out of the way
                if the other foot is not in the basin
    Keeping at least some physical contact with your friend
        place some soap in your hands
        and then lather the foot
                maybe even half way up the calf

As in all soap-and-water bathing
        almost any stroke feels exquisite
    So it is very easy to make up strokes as you go
    If you wish to follow a pattern
        use foot massage strokes
    Continue to use lavish amounts of soap
        and enough water to keep the bubbles

You can bathe and massage one foot
        easily for fifteen minutes
    But neither rush nor prolong the ceremony
    If you are totally involved
        and connected with the bathing and your friend,
                time is no longer a reality

Since the recipient is usually quite relaxed
                by the time you begin stroking
            there is little likelihood of any ticklishness
    If, however, it does occur
            stroke more slowly and more firmly
    And if the ticklishness should still remain
            discontinue the bathing
                There are other possible nurturing ceremonies

When ready
            return the foot to the basin
    Rinse the calf and foot
            by cupping and pouring water with one or both hands

At this point
            you can either remove the foot and dry it
            or if the basin contains both feet
                leave the first foot in
                while soaping and massaging the second
    Adding some hot water (carefully!)
            might be desirable now

Drying Off

Use a dry towel for the following

Encompassing the whole foot with the towel
        move the hands over the towel like this:
            up and down
            back and forth
            and in small circles
    Sliding the towel over the skin can be an exciting contrast
        but for many the sensation
                is too rough for the mood

For the toes
            there is a special treat
    Slip a folded edge of a towel
            in between a set of toes
    Then slide it gently upward for several inches

After the toes
            take this towel or preferably a separate dry towel
                and snugly wrap the foot

Once you have wrapped both feet
            place one hand on each foot

Gradually squeeze to a medium firmness
and hold a short while
When you feel ready
release very slowly
— even slowly enough
that your friend is not able to discern
when your hands have actually left contact

Afterward, perhaps continue to sit in meditation
or curl up to rest on the floor

When your friend returns to the verbal world
be open to hearing and sharing tender feelings
for each other

7 Temple of the Spirit
Massage

Hands listening
        to contours and moods
Hands dancing
        suggesting to let go
                to feel
Hands singing pleasures long forgotten

More important
        than the techniques
                is
        your own personal expression

More important than
        your own personal expression
                is
        the recipient's wishes

More important than
        the recipient's wishes
                is
        your never forcing yourself

Yet
        be open to discovering
        new horizons

It's a delicate dance

THE MASSAGE

For an extensive massage
　　　　　consult *Tantric Massage*
　　　　　　　　Volume I of *The Essential Tantra*
　　　For a simpler
　　　　　　　though equally as nurturing massage,
　　　　　explore the following strokes
　　　　　　　adapting to individual variations and circumstances,
　　　　　　　including strokes with which you are already familiar

Initially, a massage
　　　　　may be mainly a practice of strokes
　　　The learning time will vary
　　　　　for each person
　　　Be gentle with yourself
　　　　　in coordinating your mind, nervous system, and muscles
　　　　　　　into some very new patterns
　　　The gift is worth the perseverance

The following strokes can be adapted
　　　to a massage table
　　　　　or to a floor or bed massage
　　　There is, however, no necessity
　　　　　to massage the whole body
　　　　　　　every time you touch
　　　　　A neck or foot massage just by itself
　　　　　　　could be exactly what is needed

Regarding the degree of pressure
　　　　　a massage in a sensual pleasuring ceremony
　　　　　usually is one of long, flowing movements
　　　　　　　with a gentle touch
　　　A heavier pressure, athletic massage
　　　　　might be desirable for other occasions
　　　When in doubt about the pressure
　　　　　lighter might be better
　　　The recipient's preference, however,
　　　　　is the best guide

Guidelines

There are three simple guidelines
　　　　　for making touch ceremonially sensual

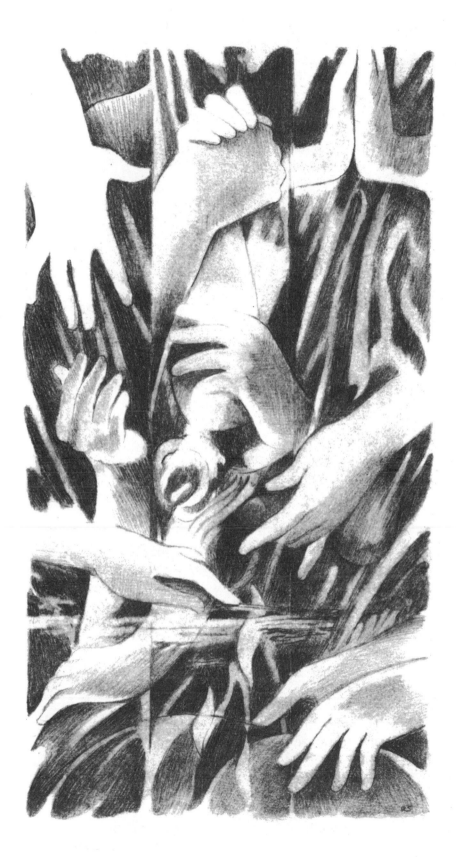

First and foremost
> be present
Letting go of expectations of the future
>> and comparisons with the past
be here now

Secondly, for most strokes
> maintain full-hand contact
>> whenever possible
Allow the palms, fingers, and thumbs
> to outline the contours

Thirdly, maintain a continuous flow
> Movements blend together
>> each one enhancing the preceding
>>> and preparing the next

Following these guidelines
> will bring a special touch to your ceremony
Allowing your hands to move intuitively
> you can open doors to inner peace

Here are a few reminders

If the sensation feels good to the recipient
> you are doing it correctly
>> — regardless of what theory or instructions might direct

Vary the pressure, tempo, and rhythm
> Repeating a stroke in the exact same way each time
>> becomes boring very quickly
>> to both the recipient and the giver

Glide on and off
> To begin a touch
>>> rather than plopping on,
>> glide on with a slow descent
>>> in the direction that your hands will be moving
> In coming off
>> continue the movement in a gradual ascent
Generally, minimize landings and take offs

If there are two of them
> massage both
For example
> stroking the left leg only and not the right
> will leave the recipient feeling very unbalanced
However,
> just the head or just the feet are fine

Minimize the talking
       An important exception
               is when the recipient needs to communicate
               deep feelings

Become centered
       Nervousness or excessive excitement
               can distract
       Tuning into and slowing your breath
               you can quieten yourself
       Being centered
               you will experience more deeply
                       your own pleasure as well

PREPARATIONS

Where?

Anywhere
               as long as distractions and interruptions are minimized
       Inside or outside is fine
               When outside
                       take precautions for insects and excessive sun
               When inside
                       unplug the phone
       If the ceremony is in a home
               arrange for all household members, including children
               not to interrupt

It is very important
               to maintain a warm temperature
       This may mean using a portable heater
               or covering parts of the recipient's body
                       not being massaged at the moment

When?

Perhaps celebrate
               a special time
       Sometimes you can be spontaneous

For an extensive ceremony
setting aside a specific day or evening
is often more conducive

With What?

Basically all you need is oil
either in a plastic squeeze bottle or a bowl
a towel or two
and a comfortable spot for the recipient to lie down

If you anticipate using feathers
or other tactile stimulators
have them close at hand

Massage tables are great
and tabletops padded with foam or blankets are fine
Make sure the table is sturdy
Otherwise, a padded floor, a bed
or the ground covered with cloth
is quite suitable
The beach
is fantastic when the sand is not a nuisance

For the covering cloth
select a sheet or other cloth
that is OK to be oiled
Some fabrics are difficult to clean
and the oil smell may not wash out

When lying on her front side
the recipient may need
a covered foam pad or a couple of rolled towels
placed under the front of the ankles
When she is lying on her back
if there is strain in her lower back
place the same pad underneath the knees

If you select a large bed
it is advantageous to have the recipient's head
at a corner at the foot of the bed
while her feet are pointing diagonally
toward the opposite corner
This allows you better access
to both the right and left sides

Perhaps use music, candle light or colored lights
incense, scented oils, flowers

          interior design of the room
          or whatever creates a comfortable ambiance
However, you do not have to create
             an extravagant environment
          every time you wish to pleasure another
Sometimes the only preparations necessary
          are to close the door
             and turn down the lights

Before Beginning

Everything ready?
        Oil, phone unplugged
            temperature warm enough
            recipient's contact lenses removed (if necessary)
            your hands warmed

Before beginning
          it is good to ask
          if there are any injuries or tender places
And remember to ask
          if anything would be particularly pleasing
Check for other possible relevancies
          such as oil in hair or time limitations

Once the recipient lies down
          invite her to take a few fuller breaths
            and to close her eyes

THE STROKES

The following set of strokes
          can be learned
            with almost no practice
They can be combined and adapted
          to almost any part of the body
Modify, use your intuition,
          use other strokes
            with which you are already familiar

Laying On Of Hands

Especially to begin, to end the massage

As an autumn leaf in slow motion
      allow your hands to come to rest
            on your beloved

Be present
      Just BE

When you feel complete
            perhaps a minute or so later
      slowly
            allow your hands to ascend
                also in slow motion

Both hands on the forehead
            Both hands on the feet
            One hand on the abdomen, the other on the forehead
            One on the sacrum, the other on the lower neck
      More important than the location
            is your presence

Chapter 9 presents more details
      under *Laying On Of Hands*

Feathering

Alternating your hands
      gracefully caress
            the surface of the recipient's skin

Short strokes, long strokes
      The pads of your fingertips
            delicately touch
                sharing subtle pleasures

Anointing With Oil

Apply the oil
      to your hands first
    With circular movements
      warm the oil
            as you spread the oil all around your hands

Now anoint your partner
using strokes similar
to the following Palm Pulling and Squeezing & Sliding

Apply the oil
to just the section you are about to massage
or if you are using a massage table,
to one whole side of the body

Palm Pulling

Especially for the sides of the torso and hips,
the inner and outer sides of the thighs

Reach across your partner
and applying full contact with your palms and fingers
firmly but gently
pull with a sliding motion
across the skin and muscles beneath
Be careful when reaching to begin each stroke
not to pinch the skin against the table/mattress beneath

Squeezing & Sliding

Especially for the arms and fingers,
the legs and the feet

Here your thumb is on one side
and your fingers are on the other side
of an appendage
Give a gentle squeeze
and slide down and off

On the arm, leg, or foot
alternate your hands
so there is a continuous contact:
As one hand lifts up to begin again
the other continues sliding

On the fingers
use only one hand
allowing your fingers to encircle the recipient's finger
and then slide off

Drumming

Especially for the back, buttocks, and backs of thighs

Rest your palm on the recipient
> while the other, closed hand
>> drums a primordial beat
>>> for several minutes or longer
>> on the back side of the flat hand
> Vary the tempo and the rhythm

Circling

Especially for the face

Applying a light pressure
> with the flat pads of your thumb
>> or the flat pads of your fingers held closely together,
> make circular movements

Most of the touch is with enough pressure
> to slide the recipient's skin
>> over the muscles beneath

At the end of the massage
> allow your beloved
>> to remain in bliss
> After a few minutes
>> being very careful not to disturb or intrude
> perhaps cuddle up beside

If it is suiting
> tuck your ceremonial guest into bed
>> and read a bedtime story
>>> to complete the Secret Garden Ceremony

Perhaps then with Spoon Breathing (see Chapter 9)
> drift into astral-land

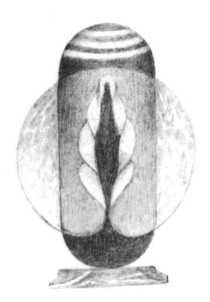

Tantric
Explorations

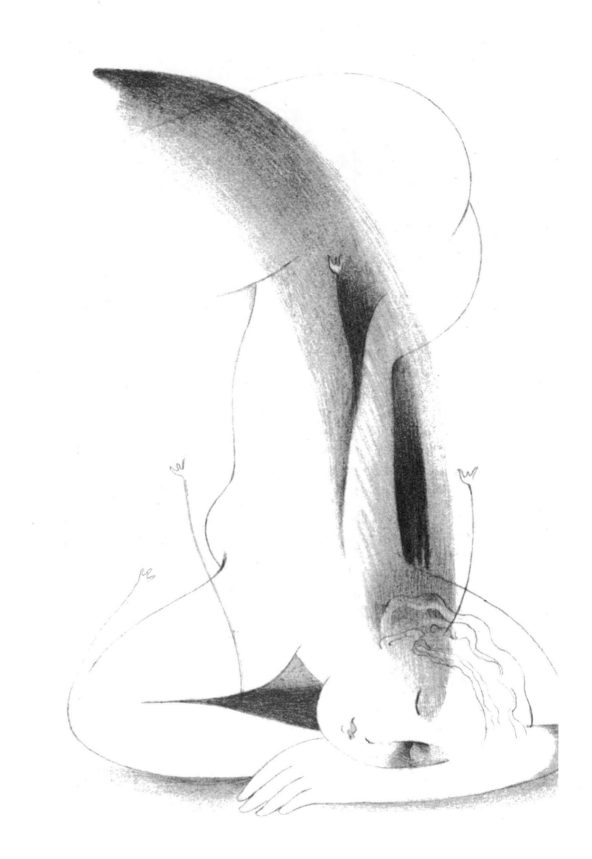

8 Equanimity
Solo Meditations

_____

Self-nurturing
　　　　is a gift of pleasure to ourself
　　This is where
　　　　sensuality, sexuality, and spirituality begin
　　　　　　—with ourself

An inner peace comes from realizing
　　　　that we already have it all within us
　　　　that it is possible to soar by ourself
　　Then when we are
　　　　with another out of a want to share
　　　　　　rather than out of a need to possess or control
　　　　there will be no strings of attachment
　　　　　　to bind and restrain

The following meditations/exercises/processes
　　　　are valuable for developing
　　　　　　a deeper appreciation of our senses
　　The focus is on relaxation
　　　　on stimulation of subtle energies
　　　　and on connection with our sensations/feelings

What is gained
　　　　enriches how we express our love to another
　　　　　　—in a sensual ceremony
　　　　　　　and in daily life

Explore and feel

THE BREATH

The breath is essential to life
and to the celebration of life
Play with these breathing meditations
Find which are most suitable
for your individual inclinations

The Equal Breath

For some the Equal Breath is one of the simplest and most effective ways to create relaxation. You can either be sitting or lying down anywhere. It requires only about ten minutes of having not to place your attention on anything in particular.

First find a beat that will function as a metronome. Close your eyes and turn inward to find the heart beat sensation. If that is not perceptible, look for any pulsation in your body. And if you find none count an even beat in your mind.

Next measure the duration of your inhalation and exhalation by counting the number of beats in each. Usually, though not always, the inhalation and exhalation will be of different durations.

Now modify your breathing pattern to equalize the number of beats of the inhalation and the exhalation. The length of the two sets is not important as long as they are equal. If there is any discomfort, you might lengthen or shorten both sets.

Continue the Equal Breath meditation for about ten or more minutes. Five or less minutes may not be long enough to be beneficial. (If necessary set an alarm rather than watching a clock).

A Variation

Continuing with the Equal Breath, gradually lengthen the duration of both sets of beats. Once you have settled into a comfortable baseline equalization, you can add two beats to both the inhalation and the exhalation. After a few minutes, add two more beats. If there is any feeling of strain, simply subtract two beats, still maintaining the equal duration. As you feel ready, continue increasing the duration by two beats about two or three more times.

Both the Equal Breath and its variation are excellent for calming yourself in a stressful situation. They are unobtrusive and can thus be practiced easily even in public.

Ocean Breath

This is an extremely powerful breathing pattern. It is wonderful for massaging the abdominal organs and often places us in a very deep state of relaxation. This exercise will require lying down approximately twenty to thirty minutes without interruptions. If the air is chilly, you might want to cover yourself before beginning.

This is a double series of twenty-one breaths. In the first series, start with an easy, normal breathing. Make each succeeding inhalation fuller than the previous one. By the twenty-first inhalation you are at your maximum inhalation.

On the second series of twenty-one, reverse the pattern. Starting with the maximum inhalation, make each succeeding inhalation less full than the preceding one until you are back to your easy breathing by the twenty-first.

As you go along, you will be approximating each increasing or decreasing increment of inhalation. Adjust in progress as necessary. If you lose your count, simply estimate.

This pattern is named the *ocean* breath since the inhalation looks like an ocean wave rolling in: It fills up first at the pelvic floor and rolls up the abdomen, up the chest, and on up to the neck. In the first few breaths, however, the ocean-like movement will not be obvious.

To exhale, simply let go and let the breath flow or rush out on its own. Do not contract the chest or abdominal muscles.

To make certain the inhalation expands in both the lower abdomen and the chest, you can rest a palm on each area.

It is very, very important not to rush any of the breaths. When your body has plenty of oxygen, it may be several seconds after an exhalation before you feel any inclination to inhale again. Allow that pause. Here lies one of the secrets to experiencing a very sensuous pleasure: Allow yourself to sink deeply into the subtle vibrations of the pause. Like a humming bird tasting the nectar of a flower, in the stillness of the pause, place your attention into your inner sensations and enjoy.

After the double series of twenty-one breaths, lie quietly and immerse yourself in the wonderful energies you have generated. This would be an excellent time for Expanding Sensations, a meditation which follows shortly.

Initially, perhaps try this exercise once a day for three or four days to get a feel for it. Then use it whenever you wish.

Heart-to-Hand Breath

This meditation is for energizing your hands and sensitizing them to tactile stimulation. You accomplish this by combining your breathing with a visualization.

Sitting or standing with your eyes closed, bring your hands up to about the height of your heart with the palms facing each other and about six inches apart. Your elbows are at your sides and your shoulders are relaxed. It is important that you are relaxed in this position. The breathing is easy and normal though it is fine if it is fuller than usual.

Now combine the breathing with this visualization: When you inhale, imagine the breath coming into your heart center from all directions—above, below, from in front, from behind, from the sides. Then with the exhalation, imagine the breath flowing outward from the heart through the shoulders, through the arms and out the hands.

Repeat this twenty-five to fifty times. The more the repetitions, the more energy you may generate.

You can use the Heart-To-Hand Breath before a laying on of hands, a massage, and specifically the following Energy Sensing.

Energy Sensing

Immediately following a Heart-to-Hand Breath, explore the energy field surrounding the body. Here the hands are very sensitive sensing devices.

With your eyes closed, very slowly separate and move your palms back and forth toward each other about an inch. They are not to touch yet. You might imagine your hands as tall grass near the ocean, the breezes gently swaying them back and forth.

Now bring your hands to a stillness, move them together about an inch, and come to a stillness again.

Next very slowly move one hand up, while the other moves down. Then reverse and continue. As your palms move past each other, tune into any sensations of magnetic pulling together or pushing apart. Again bring the hands to a stillness, move them together another inch or so, and come to a stillness again.

Now move them around each other. Continue to be open to sensing warmth and coolness, pushing and pulling tendencies, and other tinglings or hummings in or around the hands. Still avoid any physical touching. Since your eyes are closed, however, the hands might touch occasionally. Once more bring the hands to a stillness with palm facing palm.

Now very, very slowly move your palms together. Experience not knowing when your hands will touch. Be aware of the moment before they touch, the moment that they touch, and the moment after they touch.

Then very gracefully let the hands stroke each other.

After a minute or so, gently caress your face. Notice the delicate sensations.

Be open to any appreciation of your body.

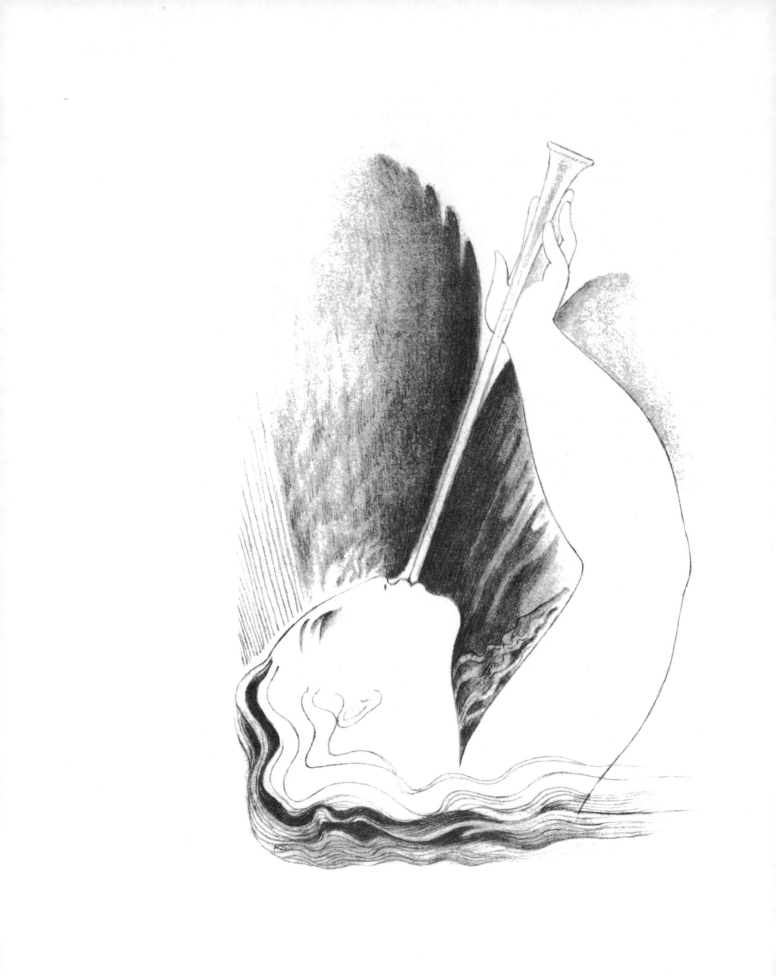

EXPANDING SENSATIONS

The secret
> of shifting from calisthenics to *sensual meditations*
> > is this:
> Immerse your awareness in a sensation
> Then imagine the sensation expanding
> > from its center outward
> > > throughout your whole body and energy field

These instructions are simple
> To follow them is not easy
Expanding Sensations requires
> an integration of mind and body
It is as if we place our whole being
> in the center of a sensation
In a sense, we become it

> We accomplish this centering and expanding with a gentle concentration. However, thoughts may intrude into our awareness. We then acknowledge to the thought that it exists and return our awareness to the sensation.

> There is no necessity to stay with any one sensation. Whenever we become aware of another predominant sensation, we can bring our awareness to that sensation and expand it.

> With the first experimentations it may seem like "nothing is happening." Remember that we are exploring subtle qualities. As we relax and tune into our body more, we will begin to discover a world that we often overlook in everyday life.

> Special times for Expanding Sensations are after a breathing meditation, during and after a self-massage, and after giving or receiving a nurturing ceremony.

An Application

Generally allowing ten to fifteen minutes, lying or sitting with eyes closed, and without interruptions, take a tour through your body.

Begin at the feet and gradually come up the entire body to the top of the head.

Starting at one foot, locate a sensation and expand it for a few moments. Then allow your awareness to move up to the ankle, find another sensation, and expand it.

And so on like this:
> calf, knee, thigh, hip
> other leg similarly
> pelvic floor, mid abdomen, upper abdomen
> one side of chest, other side of chest
> one hand, wrist, forearm, elbow, upper arm, shoulder
> other arm similarly
> back of neck, throat
> jaw, cheeks, eyes, temples, forehead, center of head
> and finally the top of head

You could locate and expand one or more sensations in each section. The sections could be small or large. Be open to the possibility that the sensations that you are *locating* are often subtle.

Sometimes it is as though your awareness just stops at a place, and thus by having your attention there, you become aware of the aliveness that is already there.

This is often a delightful, sensual journey. Use it anytime you would like to calm your body/mind.

SELF-MASSAGE

In self-massage
> we re-contact
> we re-member

Self-massage is a body-appreciation ceremony
> It is for aches and pains
> It is for pleasure

You can give yourself a quickie any time, while driving the car, watching TV, or sitting in a business conference. All you do is put pressure on a point and stroke or squeeze while you are doing the other activities.

However, when we keep part of our attention on another activity, we may not reap the full benefit of the massage. When you are ready for a special treat, try a thirty- to sixty-minute ceremony of concentrated self-massage such as the following.

This structure can be modified extensively to apply to individual situations. The single most important factor is that you set aside the time for this ceremony to occur. You, in effect, make an appointment with yourself. An excellent time is before going to sleep.

Whenever and wherever you have the ceremony, be in a place that is warm, without TV and other distractions and interruptions. This may require making arrangements with household partners.

Begin, if you wish, with a bath or shower. Then settle onto a comfortable place such as your bed. Next apply a little oil or lotion to your hands. (Add more oil as necessary.)

Begin to touch yourself. To go more deeply inward, close the eyes. Never rush or be abusive with the touching. Allow an attitude of exploration. If the automatic pilot is on while squeezing here and pushing there, you will miss great benefits and joys.

The key is to continuously place your attention in the sensation created by each touch. This sensory response becomes your meditation. And rather than apply a planned sequence of strokes to your body, let your body tell you what it wants next. Sometimes you will find a place that *hurts so good.* Sometimes emotion will come up. You are always exploring. Your inner response is your compass.

There are many ways to touch yourself. Up and down, full-hand stroking connects different areas. You can make small circles with the finger and thumb pads. You can also put fair amounts of pressure with the finger or thumb pads. With this pressure, you might slide along grooves between the muscles or bones. When applying a lot of pressure, move slowly.

Gently pounding with the fists, tapping with the fingertips, or slapping with your palms are great for stimulation. And light feather strokes with your fingertips or nails are a delight.

Mix these strokes as you desire. Lingering at some places, just stroking over others, allow the massage to unfold itself.

Sometimes you may select only one section, such as your face. Or if you want to massage your whole body, the feet are generally a good starting place. Be sure to include inside the ears, under the arms, the genitals, perhaps inside the mouth and the nose.

Once you complete the self-massage, rest and Expand Sensations. It is almost like two massages — the first with the hands, the second with the mind.

Then if you go to sleep for the night after this, notice how your body feels the next morning.

Until we can truly appreciate
      our own body and senses
we may find that instead of pleasuring another
      we are only acting out a boring routine

If ceremony is to have meaning
      it is to come out of our own aliveness
If we are to celebrate
      we must truly appreciate the vehicle
         through which we experience our celebration

9 Energy Dance
Mutual Meditations

Striving for pleasure
        prevents tasting the subtle nectars
    Grasping,
        we can not experience the gentle vibrations
           of love, joy, and inner peace

This chapter like the previous
        is about becoming more aware
           of the subtle qualities of pleasure
           and developing a sense of ceremony
    In the previous chapter
        we soared solo
    Here we join with a partner

None of the meditations/exercises/processes/games
        require dexterity or practice
    Simply enter with a willingness
        to allow the sensations and feelings
           to unfold as you give and as you receive
    Choose a meditation that interests you and your partner
        and explore

Relax
    Linger
        Discover

MAPPING

One of the greatest inhibitors
              to the experience of pleasure
      is our comparative mind
We assume that we know
      what our partner likes
              (which often is really a projection
                  of what we like)
And relying on our past experiences
      we also assume that we know what we like now
Unfortunately, our assumptions
      are not always correct
Mapping is a meditation to check our assumptions
      and to discover new sensual realms

In Mapping, as in land surveying, we discover the highs and lows. It also serves as an important communication tool which can be adapted to any nurturing situation.

The form of the communication is like this: with a range of "plus three" to "minus three," we indicate the degree of desirability or undesirability of each sensation.

The communication can be verbal or manual. With the latter, one hand is the plus hand and the other is the minus hand. Displaying one, two, or three fingers indicates the degree. For zero, the neutral point, form a circle with the positive hand's thumb and index finger.

It is very important to remember Mapping is a rating of the sensation, not of the performance of the mapper. Also, there is a tendency for the neutral point to shift throughout the process. Since this is not a scientific study, allow this subjective variability to be OK.

Whole Body Mapping

To begin, the recipient lies front down. She/he can be nude or minimally clothed.

As the mapper, you initiate the touches on the upper back and map down to the feet. Then softly invite your partner to turn over. Here begin the mapping at the feet and come up the legs, torso, arms, and finally the neck and head.

There are some guidelines to follow in this Whole Body Mapping.

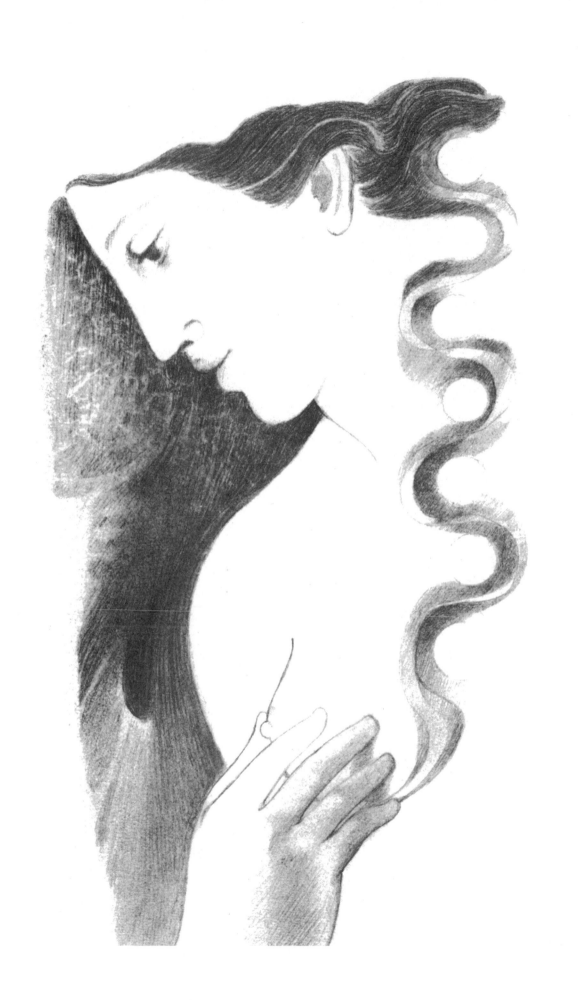

Touch simply.

Touch only one location at a time.

And touch only small areas about six inches being maximum. When the touch is much longer, there might be a "plus two" at one part and a "minus one" at another.

Vary the direction, pressure, and type of touch.

If there is a minus response, avoid repeating that particular touch on that part of the body. Equally important, let go of any performance of giving your partner a "plus three."

For right now at least, you are surveying. A massage can come later.

Sometimes until a mapper has had a personal experience of being mapped, she/he might find it a little boring. Keep in mind that this is a valuable service to the recipient. It is also a great way to *turn on / tune in* the whole body.

Once a giver and receiver become familiar with the plus-three-to-minus-three method, Mapping feedback can be shared in any pleasuring experience as an occasional communication.

GAMES

Approach the next meditations
as gentle games
They vary from quiet movements
to delightful play
to energizing massages
Which one you choose
would depend on the mood

Rag Doll

This is a simple and beautiful meditation
teaching about letting go and surrender

For us to be able to truly receive a gift from another
  we must be able to surrender
In surrender
    we choose
        to be where we are
This is in contrast to submission
      in which we *give in* or *give up*
          to another's power
            because we think we have no alternative

In this meditation
      the recipient is a rag doll
thus, no thoughts
      no expectations
      no comparisons
      and no muscular tension

As the giver, you approach the rag doll with *beginner's mind.* This is the first time you have ever seen a rag doll, and in your fascination, you want to discover what it is like. Exploring from this perspective, you might come to a wonderful, new appreciation of your partner.

Your discovery takes the form of randomly and slowly moving the recipient's arms, legs, and head. Sometimes there are gentle stretches. This is all done nonverbally and without rushing.

The recipient may have a tendency to help in lifting the limbs or to hold on to the muscles. If you notice this, softly invite her/him to take a fuller breath and upon exhaling to relax the muscles. If this breathing technique is ineffective, it is better to silently allow the recipient to remain tense than to try to verbally or manually force a relaxation.

First, invite the recipient to lie down and to close her/his eyes. Then select either arm to begin the meditation. Slowly and gently explore all possible movements in the fingers, wrist, elbow, and shoulder area.

After the first arm, continue for about five minutes on each appendage in a similar fashion with the other arm, then one leg, and then the other. On the legs, support the knee joint when lifting and lowering a bent leg so as to avoid *popping* the knee when you straighten the leg.

Next take your friend on a *space walk* by lifting and slowly moving both legs.

After lowering the legs, introduce similar lifting movements very slowly to the head and neck.

When you are ready, gracefully slide your fingers off the ends of the hair strands.

And to complete, letting your fingers be like feathers, gently slide your fingertips from the top of her/his head down off the fingertips. Then slide from the top of the head down off the tips of the toes.

What may be the most important part of this meditation is the experience following the movements. The slow and gentle movements have stimulated subtle sensations, and the recipient, most likely, is deeply relaxed.

Rest in silence
    until your partner feels like coming back to Earth

Born Again

As with the Rag Doll
    this meditation teaches
        about letting go and surrender
    In Born Again
        it is as if you were a flower bud opening
          to the warming light of the sun

Here the recipient, perhaps with shoes off, lies on one side and tenses up into a tight fetal position. Holding this tension for about ten seconds, she/he might recontact what *holding on* feels like. Then, remaining in the fetal position, she/he simply relaxes.

Now with palms and fingers, stroke gently every section of the recipient's body. As you do this, very, very gradually uncoil the contracted form. Focus much more on the stroking than on the unfolding.

Eventually your partner is lying flat on her/his back with the arms at the sides.

Take a final visual check to make sure there are no curves in the alignment.

Then give a feather stroke from the head down off the fingers and from the head down off the toes.

Silently relax as the recipient floats.

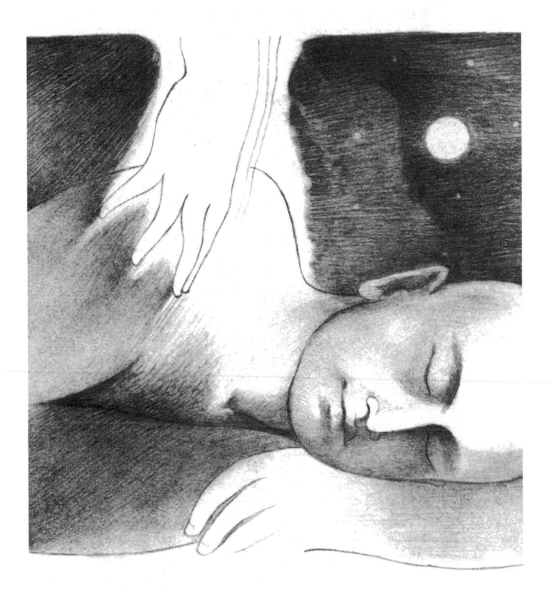

Bliss Caress

This would be a blissful follow-up
        after a Whole Body Mapping
        which would have already sensitized the skin surface

You can use one or more of these:
      feathers, especially ostrich or peacock
      silk scarves
      furry fabrics
      your hair or beard
      brushes (be gentle if the bristles are hard)
      plastic wrap
      possibly your breath
      your fingertips

        For about five to twenty minutes, caress your partner by making long, flowing strokes all over her/his nude or partially nude body.

The number of substances is not important,
      the gentle, connecting touches are.

Grooming

In this delightful meditation we are borrowing from our furry cousins' grooming behaviors. And since we can use powder here, Grooming is an alternative to oil massage.

First, add a powder, such as corn starch, over all of one side of your nude or partially nude partner. Sprinkling the powder like gentle rain creates a special sensation in itself. (If no powder is available, you can still do this meditation.)

Then *groom* your friend with rapid hand movements in the following manner. With your thumb on one side and the fingers on the other side of a section of skin, rapidly and gently squeeze them together and lift up. The hands alternate with each other in rapid succession. In some areas, such as the thighs, you will probably see a ripple effect on the skin.

Gradually go up and down both sides of the recipient's body. On the face, throat, breasts, and genitals, be very gentle and a little slower.

If your hands become tired, you can slow down or feather stroke with your fingertips for a while.

A nice addition after Grooming is to caress your partner with about two feet of plastic wrap. Slide the edge across the skin. Notice how it statically clings to the skin.

Hair Brushing

Perhaps sitting in the sun or by a fireplace
          slowly brush or comb through your partner's hair
If you wish to be more elaborate
          you could shampoo first

Maybe lullaby or hum
      as you brush

Slap Happy

This is *the energizer.* It is fantastic after driving or traveling for many hours or when you need to wake up.

Before beginning, the giver removes rings and watch; the recipient, any dangling earrings.

Then the standing recipient spreads her/his feet about shoulder distance apart and bends forward at the waist. It is best to let the knees bend a little and let the head and arms dangle toward the floor.

Now as the giver, *slap* your friend into a happy state. Standing from behind, begin slapping on the muscles on each side of the spine. It is usually best to totally avoid the bony part of the spine. Use the fleshy part of the little-finger side of your hands. You can also use the palms slightly cupped or the little-finger sides of your fists. It is best to alternate the hands: one goes down while the other goes up.

The amount of pressure on different parts of the body will vary from person to person. Be on the conservative side until the recipient indicates that more intensity is preferable.

After the back, slap with your palms on one leg at a time. Do this all the way down to the toes and back up. On the legs both hands can slap at the same time rather than in an alternating manner. Also be very careful to avoid the scrotum. In this bent-over position, the scrotum is much closer to your hands than you might imagine.

Next slap on the back area until you come to the arms.

On each arm, follow a similar pattern as on the legs.

Return to the back, this time standing at the recipient's head. Now focus on the upper back and shoulders. Gradually move to the scalp. Here briskly slide your finger pads back and forth but without much pressure. Increase the speed for a bit. Then suddenly lift your hands off. Voilà! The sudden ending is a sweet energetic thrill.

ENERGY

In a sensual ceremony
> many subtle vibratory qualities
> come to consciousness
The following meditations
> aid in recognizing these qualities

To explore energy
> it is best to enter with a relaxed attentiveness
> and a willingness to try something new

Spoon Breathing

In Spoon Breathing
> we combine touch with unison breathing
This is an especially intimate way
> to share some quiet moments together
Try beginning or ending a ceremony this way

First your partner lies down on her/his side with the knees pulled forward a little for balance. Then also on your side, snuggle in closely behind. Your lower arm can be pointing upward, perhaps with a pillow or a folded towel placed between the arm and the head. If this position is uncomfortable, place your lower arm between yourself and your partner. Your upper arm rests on your partner's upper arm.

It is important not to tense the muscles by holding your partner. Simply relax and let your bodies melt together.

Once you become comfortable, tune into and follow your partner's breathing, matching the inhalation and the exhalation. This may at first seem awkward, but usually after a minute or so, it becomes natural.

For the purposes of this meditation, your partner can breathe in one of two ways. The first is to breathe as usual without any attempted alteration of pace or volume. The second method is to take slower and fuller breaths. This latter pattern seems more likely to enhance the experience of deep relaxation and subtle energy flows. Either way can be enjoyable.

Without watching the time, you might try this for ten minutes or longer. If sleep occurs, allow it. And if anything becomes a strain or a hassle, forget about the breathing and lie there cuddling.

Aura Massage

Here we bring our attention
        to the energy fields around the recipient's physical body
Sometimes referred to as an aura
        these energy fields are quite subtle
When we are calm and centered
        we are more likely to become aware of them

Heart-to-Hand Breath

While it is not necessary to begin an aura massage with the Heart-to-Hand Breath, starting this way is an excellent preparation.

With your eyes closed, sitting or standing behind your reclining partner's head, bring your hands up to about the height of your heart.

Your palms are facing each other, about six inches apart. Your elbows are at your sides and your shoulders are relaxed.

When you inhale, imagine the breath coming into your heart center from all directions. In the exhalation, imagine the breath flowing from the heart to the shoulders, to the arms, and out the hands.

Repeat this combined breathing and visualization for twenty-five to fifty breaths.

By the end of this breathing meditation, you are more likely to have an inner calmness and your hands feel energized.

Energy Sensing

Next bring your hands from about six inches to one-half inch above your partner's head. Be careful not to physically touch the skin as that would be a predominating sensation.

Now slowly move your hands above the surface, using them as sensing devices. *Listen* with them. There might be humming, tingling, magnetic pushing or pulling, warmth or coolness. These may vary over different locations.

A slower movement is often necessary to become aware of the subtle vibrations. And you may find that the backs of your hands are a little more sensitive to sensing the different qualities of energy.

Continue the sensing around your partner's head and any other part of the body for several minutes before beginning the aura massage. (Actually you have already been massaging the aura, though your attention has initially been on your own sensing.)

An Aura Massage

Still without touching the physical body, begin to massage the energy field. There are several theories about what to do with this energy. For our purposes here, we allow ourself to be like a child again and pretend. Here simply play.

Move your hands as if you are polishing or combing the energy field. You can fluff it up or swirl it. Still moving slowly enough to sense the energy, allow your intuition or imagination to guide you. If you are willing to pretend, this can be a fun experience.

Maybe play with the aura massage for five to thirty minutes.

Afterward remain silent and allow the recipient to relax.

Whenever she/he returns to the physical world, share with each other about the experiences.

LAYING ON OF HANDS

Laying on of hands is an ancient ritual
    While most often associated
                      with healing and religious rites
               it is also a valuable part of sensual ceremonies
    A touch that is still
                  and that conveys presence
           can communicate feelings of love and care
                far more deeply than most words

How we lay our hands
                 is more important
                     in this meditation
              than *where*
Actually, *resting on of hands*
               is a more accurate denotation

When you begin a laying on of hands, you might imagine that your hands are like an autumn leaf, descending in slow motion to rest on the earth. The autumn leaf has no expectations. It is not in a hurry. When it touches the earth, all it can do is rest there—simply be there.

To complete a laying, reverse this process, also in slow motion.

Entering and leaving the energy field in this manner is a nonverbal way of asking permission. It indicates a reverence. If we allow ourself to be as the autumn leaf without demands and without performance, we will nourish a deep sense of trust and connection.

You can give a whole *massage* with just a series of laying on of hands. Or you can add them as a part of a more inclusive nurturing meditation. One to five minutes in each position is usually sufficient.

Helmet

From behind the recipient's head, rest your palms so that your thumbs are side by side with the thumb pads on the middle of the forehead and your fingers are on the temples.

The helmet is also an especially nurturing way to begin a facial massage.

Third Eye and Navel

The *third eye* refers to an area approximately in the center of the forehead just above the eyebrows. Often we can feel a concentrated energy here.

While at your partner's side, make both of your hands into a relaxed fist shape. Then extend your thumbs, one toward the third eye, the other toward the navel. Very, very slowly allow your thumbs to descend to about a quarter inch above the third eye and navel.

Perhaps after about thirty seconds there, allow them to lightly touch the skin beneath.

Abdomen and Forehead

From beside your reclining partner, lay one of your palms over the third eye area and the other palm over the abdomen, a couple of inches below the navel. You might find that the energy flows more intensely when the palm's center is over the body's midline.

Tantric Laying On Of Hands

Here your awareness focuses on your middle fingers even though your whole palm touches.

Your upper hand rests so that the palm is on the recipient's forehead and your middle finger is at the center top of the head. This place was a fontanel, or *soft spot,* when we were babies.

Your other hand rests so that your middle finger touches the perineum, the area just between the anus and genitals. You may first need to separate your partner's thighs a little. Then if necessary, you would first use your upper hand to lift the scrotum and penis so that your lower hand can be in fuller contact with the pelvic floor.

As in the rest of this series, your hands are simply resting in place rather than applying pressure or movement.

Feet

Standing or sitting at your partner's feet, rest your fingers on top of the feet while your thumbs curve around, inside, to the underside in the arches.

This is also a wonderful way to conclude a full body massage.

These are only five specific positions
        from many possibilities
    Explore any intuitive inclination
    And remember that your attentiveness
            is more important
                    than where you actually touch

CHANTING

Chanting can nurture
    Chanting can stimulate
            subtle energies

Which chant you use
        is not important for these meditations
Any syllable or series of soothing syllables
        is perfect
As a suggestion
        try *OM* or *AUM*

There are at least two ways you can use chanting in a sensual ceremony. Either could open or close a ceremony or be a whole ceremony.

Together

The first is to chant in conjunction with your partner.

Here you sit closely and facing your partner. It might be helpful to have eyes closed to eliminate visual distractions. After being aware of your breathing for a minute or so, begin to chant together.

The chant itself could be continuous, each taking a breath when necessary. Or you could chant and then inhale in unison with your partner.

The intention here is to merge the sounds and energies. After a period of time, perhaps twenty minutes or longer, there may be a sense of Oneness.

Solo

Almost as if lullabying, you chant as your partner reclines beside you. This can be a very nurturing moment.

Here the chant might be melodic rather than a single tone. If you are not accustomed to chanting or singing in front of another, it might be a little scary at first. How well you are chanting, however, is not important. What is important is that you are truly sharing yourself.

When to chant is often an intuitive choice. One special time is when pouring water on your partner in a bath. Another is at the ending of a massage.

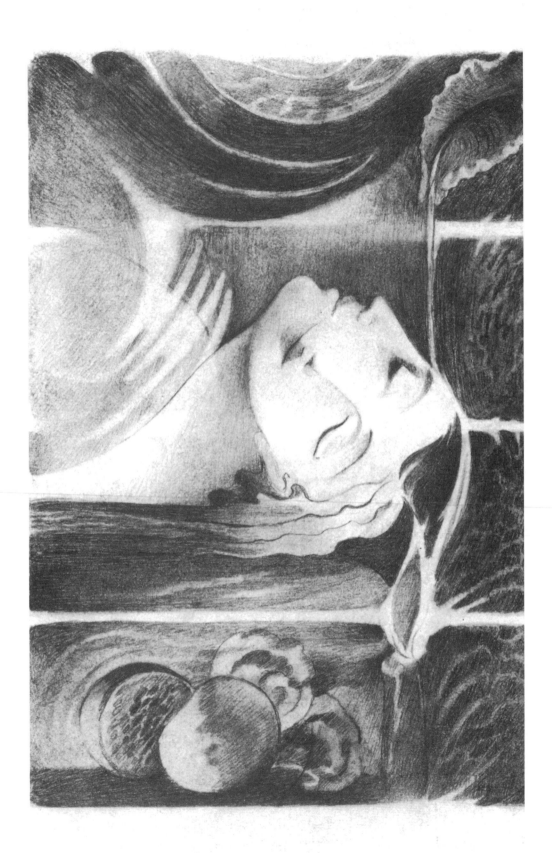

The willingness to experiment
           is the key to these meditations
    When we discover
           our ability to experience subtle vibratory qualities
                within each sensation and each feeling
           our relationship to our body and our partner
                will be immensely enriched

The *tantric explorations*
           of these last two chapters
           are valuable preparations for the Secret Garden Ceremony
    They are special means for rediscovering
           ourself and our partner

To be able to experience pleasure
           in a way that neither craves nor condemns the body
                is a celebration

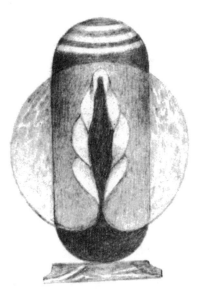

EPILOGUE

While techniques and suggestions
        provide practical guidelines,
    they are still only guidelines.
They are form,
    not essence.

When we open
    to inner beauty,
When we bring
       presence to our self-expression,
    we approach essence.

Michelangelo once was asked
    why God favored him with such special talent
    to sculpt forms into marble.

Michelangelo responded
    it was not his talent
    to sculpt into the stone.
Rather,
    his mastery
       was in the ability

to see the beauty
  that God had already created
    in the marble.

Michelangelo would then simply uncover
  that beauty
    by smoothing away the rough edges.

In tantric sensual ceremony
  we bring our attention
    to sensory and feeling experiences.
  We slow down
    so that we become aware of subtleties.
  We discover
    the beauty
      beneath the rough edges.
  We nurture
    the senses in gentleness.

The heart is touched
  and we experience joy.

Sacred Orgasms

SOURCES

These are the authors and teachers who have had a major influence on what I wrote in *Sacred Orgasms*.

Tantra

> Tarthang Tulku, a Tibetan lama, guided me to a deep understanding of meditation, though he spoke of sexuality only once in my presence.
>
> Jwala is an American tantrika who walks her talk.
>
> Ralph Metzner, Ph.D., in *Maps of Consciousness* was the first to present, for me, a clear picture of tantra.

Taoism

> Stephen T. Chang, M.D., Ph.D., author of *The Tao of Sexology*, through his seminars, books, and friendship, has taught me much about Taoism.
>
> The *I Ching*, by Richard Wilhelm, translated by Cary F. Baynes, would be the one book if I could keep only one.

Quodoushka

> Harley SwiftDeer Reagan, a true warrior in many senses, is a Native American shaman making available the Quodoushka teachings to those who are willing to take the leap. Diane Nightbird and Stephanie Rainbow Lighting Elk have greatly enhanced my understanding of these teachings.

Energy

> Billie Hobart, in my first seminar with her, led me in a guided meditation focusing on an energy center above my head. When my awareness touched the center, tears came, and I felt I had *come home*.

Western Sexology/Erotology

> The Institute for the Advanced Study of Human Sexuality in San Francisco provided me with teaching and learning opportunities unparalleled in any other contemporary academic setting. I am especially grateful to Clark Taylor, Ph.D., Laird Sutton, Ph.D., Marguerite Rubenstein, Ph.D., Ted McIlvenna, Ph.D., and Wardell Pomeroy, Ph.D.

Dedicated to
my energy teachers

Tarthang Tulku
Billie Hobart
Harley SwiftDeer
Carolyn Parker

A Special Acknowledgment to
Jeannie Kruger
without whom this book
would not be
what it became.

ACKNOWLEDGMENTS

Were it not for Carolyn Parker, this edition might never have been accessed.
Several dear friends and professionals gave feedback: Danielle Berrien,
Laurel Fishman, Helen Davidson, Rich Tapper, Ina Laughing Winds,
and Jake Kerr.
My appreciation likewise goes to several others who contributed in different,
special ways: Jimmy Scott, Ph.D., Stan Russell, Ph.D., and all the
people who over the years told about their out-of-the-ordinary
orgasms.

INTRODUCTION

Orgasm is at the center of the sacred circle.
Dancing in this center, we can come to know God
and all other creations
more deeply, more profoundly than by any other path.

This is the central teaching of five unincarnated companions who have invited me to include additional concepts and eight meditations not in the first edition of *Sacred Orgasms.*

In this new edition, the first two sections remain basically the same as in the first edition. In Section III, "Orgasm as Transformation," however, I am principally a translator-communicator. Yet the text is by no means a verbatim transcription of voices out of the ethers. I wish this book had been that simple. Using my personal experiences and studies of several esoteric paths, I have had a sometimes difficult, sometimes exciting challenge interpreting and conveying into written language my communications with these five beings.

For me, it all seems to be a journey to the mountaintop only to discover another, higher mountaintop in the distance. Were it not for the experiences that led to writing *Tantric Massage* and *Sensual Ceremony*, I doubt I would have discovered *Sacred Orgasms.* And a future edition of this book would no doubt be different from the current one. Nonetheless, I often write with a definitive tone. While I have no certainty this is ultimate truth, a decade of exploration suggests the following concepts are a very useful paradigm, which indeed constitutes a paradigm shift for most of us.

I encourage you to consider the teachings and to explore the eight meditation practices that follow. If they do not resonate with you, if they do not grow corn to feed you on your own unique path, drop them. But do not drop your spiritual passion. There are many paths to God.

THE COMPANIONS

I call these five unincarnated beings *companions.* While they have indeed been teachers and guides for me, they have repeatedly said that our relationship is by no means a one-way street. Being incarnated—having a physical body—allows opportunities to learn and create in ways not possible without a physical body. Unincarnated beings learn and gain from what we incarnated beings experience and accomplish.

According to these five companions, there are at least three basic types of beings: *incarnating beings, essence beings* (what some call spirit guides), and *Source* (what many term as God or Goddess).

Incarnating beings can incarnate on this planet, simplistically stated, as human beings, animals, plants, or some types of crystalline structures. Three of my five companions are currently unincarnated incarnating beings who some might designate as ascended masters. In at least one of their incarnations as a human being, they fully developed all of their *soul centers* (discussed later). This allowed perception of all forms of existence. Thus, I call them *seers.* In each of our personal journeys, seers can be immensely meaningful teachers. Becoming more consciously connected with such beings is also a likely result with the eight meditations that follow.

Essence beings, a second category, are sometimes called spirit guides or spirit companions. These are beings of light who can never incarnate. They sometimes, though, might present a semblance of some physical life form. Some essence beings are devas, of which some hold a sort of "spirit genetic code" for a specific type of physical life form.

Some other essence beings I term *energy companions.* Each incarnated human being incarnates with an energy buddy that supports and learns right along with that human for that whole incarnation.

Some would call these guardian angels, though I find such a label far too limiting. A large set of wings would probably only slow everything down, and *guarding* is a narrow concept for only one of an energy companion's many functions. *Energy modulating* for me is a more accurate characterization. A being with a physical body cannot handle some of the intensity and energy patterns from some nonphysical beings without the energy first being modified. Unlike Icarus, whose fall from the heavens when the wax on his artificial wings melted in his flight too close to the sun, our energy companions would provide an energetic shade so our physical bodies would not be overwhelmed in our more intensely connected moments with God.

Yu, a fourth companion, is the sound/thought form/name with which I refer to my personal energy companion. This is the "spirit companion" I wrote about in the beginning of the Introduction to *The Essential Tantra.* The ringing in my ear, especially when I was talking or thinking about tantra, was often this being's way at that time of encouraging me to pay attention to something that might be of particular relevance. Now Yu organizes and facilitates my communications with other unincarnated beings.

God/Source/Goddess is a third category of being, of which there is only one such being. This is the conscious central operating system of all existence, incarnated and unincarnated. I prefer the term *Source* because it suggests an originating principle and is gender neutral. However, flowing with convention, I will often write *God.*

God is a fifth companion suggesting the additional concepts and eight meditations in *Sacred Orgasms.* Given my religious upbringing, writing that I am in direct communication with God feels very presumptuous. However, such communication is entirely consistent with the eight meditations' purpose, which includes increasing the capacity of any human being's conscious self to communicate and connect with God. Thus, God is everyone's companion. The only difference is that some have clearer connections than others have.

Please realize that while I have been deeply involved in spiritual and shamanic study for a number of years, playing with beings in other realms has never been an attraction for me. I was far more interested in physical and energetic connections with physical human beings. Tantric massage and sensual ceremony were clearly my preferred cup of tea. And to be a translator-communicator rather than the sole creative intellect behind the teachings and meditations in *Sacred Orgasms* is not my fancied self-image. But my spiritual passion to know God more deeply, to dance in the Light, has led me to this role.

In the day-to-day communications, I have sometimes felt these five companions don't really comprehend or remember what it is like to cross a physical street with eighteen-wheelers bearing down on your ass from both directions. At the same time, I have experienced a wonderful, unconditional acceptance from these beings when I have ranted and raved my frustrations regarding our communications or the lack of them.

My companions have suggested I not write in this book about the meditation method through which I cognitively communicate with them. That method is unrelated to this book, and it is only one of many possible ways to be in communication with unincarnated companions. Moreover, they continue to insist that I am in communication with them in ways I do not yet comprehend.

Two factors balance my concern that my written words here might take the reader on a spiritual wild goose chase. First, in contrast to a day-to-day perspective, over the duration of the communications with these companions I have in general found unfolding in front of me an integrated esoteric cosmology that seems quite consistent.

Second, many of my experiences of the four types of orgasm delineated by the companions are very real. Many of the orgasm patterns have been repeated, sometimes in conscious meditation with myself or with others. Many have been very intense. And while the conceptual distinctions in some ways lack clarity, rarely do the orgasms.

ORGASM

To understand the concept of orgasm and the following meditations, we need a concept of anatomy not common to a physiology textbook. In *Sacred Orgasms*, a human being is the interaction between the *soul system* and the *incarnated systems*, summarized in the following outline and discussed more in the main text:

A. the soul system
- soul
- soul centers
- sphere
- core

B. the seven incarnated systems
  a.   the six subtle energy systems
      • spirit body
      the five "engine" systems
          • light body
          • chakra system
          • resonance system
          • kundalini system
          • resource system
  b.   • physical body

At some point after the joined sperm and egg attach to the uterine wall, a soul merges with the zygote. The ensuing interaction results in the development of six subtle energy systems, such as the chakras and kundalini system. These six systems are what we call life, bringing vibrancy, motility, and mobility to physical matter.

Together these six subtle energy systems and the physical body constitute what I call the incarnated systems. A human being, though, is the totality of these incarnated systems plus the soul system.

The eight meditations are called the integration meditations because their purpose is to extensively develop the ten soul centers and soul system and to integrate the soul system with the incarnated systems at a far deeper level than we are likely to in typical, everyday modern life.

Very few of the religious and physical development traditions with which I am familiar focus on developing the soul system, even though their tenets may imply this. The actual impact is primarily on the different incarnated systems, some teachings emphasizing the religious aspects in the sense of ritual practices or morality, and some teachings emphasizing the physical and energetic aspects, as in many martial arts and Olympic trainings.

To fully develop the soul system requires an immense amount of energy. Healthy food, sunlight, clean air and water, exercise, harmonious environs: All these nurture us with good energy for good health. But orgasm, more than any other human activity, provides us with the most of the kind of energy best suited for developing the soul system.

Orgasm, as conventionally understood, is a highly pleasurable, explosive-like experience with muscular contractions in the pelvic floor, often resulting from stimulation of physical places such as the penis, clitoris, G spot, or prostate. I call this physical body orgasm a *sexual orgasm,* a category that includes a wide variety of sexually orgasmic experiences, such as the often-reported distinction between a clitoral orgasm and a G-spot orgasm.

My five companions clearly communicate that sexual orgasm is but one of four major types of orgasm a human is capable of having. Two other incarnated systems and the soul system can orgasm as well. Perhaps because these three other types of orgasm may not feel sexual or may not occur in a sexual context, throughout the centuries some of these other types of orgasms may have been considered mystical experiences. In cultures where sexuality and spirituality are so hierarchically differentiated as in ours, such a mystical experience would rarely be conceptualized in the same category with sexual orgasm.

As with sexual orgasms, the three other orgasm types have tremendous variations. Conceptually, the distinctions between the four types are clear for me, but I cannot always classify my orgasmic experiences as one type or another. Some orgasms are two or more types occurring in conjunction. In most cases, these other types of orgasmic experiences do not feel sexual, at least for me. Sometimes the orgasms are subtle, sometimes very intense, sometimes without sensations I consider pleasurable. Later in this text are many examples of what I term *out-of-the-ordinary orgasms*—individuals' experiences of variations on the orgasm rainbow.

The definition of orgasm that the companions present is very abstract and easily encompasses a wide array of phenomena:

> An orgasm is an event where two or more vibratory patterns change so that they resonate with each other, and a new vibratory pattern occurs which consists of the initial vibratory patterns plus the vibratory pattern of *primordial incarnated energy.*

The key to this definition of orgasm is the primordial incarnated energy. If this type of energy is not generated/created/originated/developed, the event is not an orgasm.

An incarnated human being functions with ten types of *incarnated energy.* The primordial type is my word for undifferentiated, not-yet-formed incarnated energy. This is the easiest of the ten types of incarnated energy to be transformed into the other nine types as needed by any system for any function. And primordial incarnated energy is the type of energy needed in immense quantities to develop the soul system and to integrate it with the incarnated systems, which is the purpose of the eight meditations.

Accessing via orgasm these immense amounts of primordial incarnated energy is central to understanding *Sacred Orgasms.* In any orgasm, we generate this most utilizable form of energy available for life. Also in orgasm, we are the closest to God we can be—our energetic patterns become more like God's energetic patterns than in any other event. This is why orgasms are sacred.

Equally as important to understanding *Sacred Orgasms* is the realization that pleasure is only one of the two primary functions of orgasm. Transformation, a second function, is the primary focus in *Sacred Orgasms.* (Likewise, understanding transformation is a key to understanding tantric philosophy, as discussed in the Introduction to *The Essential Tantra.*)

When we embrace the role of orgasm in the transformation of energy, in the transformation of emotions, and in the transformation of our capacity to function via nonphysical intent, we will no longer be restricted to a paradigm where what we call sexuality and what we call spirituality are in opposition. Rather, we will find the interaction between our sexual and our spiritual desires to be a basic, natural dynamic in our existence.

THE INTEGRATION MEDITATIONS

Directly from my five companions and new with this edition of *Sacred Orgasms* are two separate sets of four meditative practices.

The four *intensification meditations* are to tonify and expand the capacity of the soul system and each of the seven incarnated systems. The four *orgasm meditations* are to have one of each of the four types of orgasms in a *very* mild form in order to generate more primordial incarnated energy.

Together the two sets are labeled the *integration meditations* because the main purpose is to integrate the soul system and the incarnated systems. While perhaps not stated quite this way in spiritual traditions, the meditations' objective seems to me to be in alignment with many core esoteric teachings.

For all but one of the meditations, all we basically need is our conscious awareness (attention), our intent, and a minimal knowledge of the anatomy of a human being as presented here. The meditations can be done individually in solitude, with a partner of the same or different sex, or with a group. An uninterrupted space is also important. Except possibly for the sexual orgasm meditation, each meditation is likely to take only one to two minutes after the initial learning.

Repeating the meditations on an ongoing basis is necessary in order to have much impact, though I have no idea if the maximum effect requires a year, several decades, or several lifetimes. My companions have not given an answer to this question.

My companions have communicated these meditation practices to me only with the agreement that I would teach the meditations to others. After I taught a few friends individually and in a few seminars, the companions added a couple of very minor modifications, based on what they perceived in the energy patterns of the people while they did the meditations.

Except for the sexual orgasm meditation, I have never seen or heard of any meditations quite like these. Fortunately, these meditations could likely be practiced along with many other meditative or spiritual practices from other traditions. A notable exception would be where masturbation or sex with another is prohibited.

ORGASM MANIFESTING

The basic idea of orgasm manifesting, or what some call sex magic, is that at the moment of orgasm the individual intends a desired goal to become manifest. The resulting energy of the orgasm is what fuels whatever is needed to accomplish the intent.

According to the companions, such orgasm manifesting is definitely *not* to be used in direct conjunction with these eight meditations. However, consensual orgasm manifesting in conjunction with sexual orgasms other than a part of the integration meditations is fine.

In the integration meditations, our soul, with its far greater wisdom than our everyday mind, knows the optimum ways to utilize the primordial incarnated energy to accomplish the purposes of the meditation. To send our orgasmic energy off in some other direction would be self-defeating.

The companions add that practicing what is sometimes termed sexual vampirism is *always* very unwise. Long-term and extensive use of such a practice can result in illness and eventually death for all parties involved. Writings and discussions of both Indian Tantra and Chinese Taoism have some references to practices where experienced practitioners will literally suck the primordial incarnated energy off the body of an often unwitting and sometimes younger person in sexual orgasm.

(Note that sexual vampirism is a conscious act and is usually different from situations where we feel drained or disturbed while being around someone in general day-to-day interactions. When another is, for example, aggressive, angry, or acting in a needy manner, the seemingly negative effect on us is likely the result of our own "stuckness." We can treat such situations as being a mirror of who we really are and explore growing beyond our own limitations. Sometimes, though, our drained or disturbed feeling is due to another's disturbing energy patterns that are not consciously intended. This topic is beyond the focus of *Sacred Orgasms* and is anticipated to be in a future book.)

Sexual vampirism is in direct contrast to the energy reciprocity that occurs naturally when lovers simply honor and celebrate each other while making love. My companions say that doing the integration meditations on an ongoing basis with a consenting, compassionate partner not only accomplishes the energy buildup desired in sexual vampirism, but does so in a way far more powerful, in far more areas of our being, and in a manner that is healthy and beneficial for all people involved.

THE CHAKRAS AND THE SOUL CENTERS

Many esoteric frameworks include something about chakras. The most popular conceptualization of this Sanskrit term is that seven subtle energy wheels/disks/vortexes exist along the core of the body between the pelvic floor and the crown of the head.

In the first edition of *Sacred Orgasms*, I did not feel confident enough to state my experience, which in some ways differed from most of the popular esoteric beliefs. When I first began the types of meditations that resulted in writing *Sacred Orgasms*, I had many experiences suggesting there are ten of something. Within a year I began studying with my shamanic teacher, who authoritatively said there are ten principal chakras, the additional three being above the head. Within two years I learned from an esoteric meditation teacher a specific ten-chakra meditation.

I encourage you to approach with an open mind the following anatomy of a being. In this framework, there are ten principal chakras and ten soul centers along the core of the body from the pelvic floor to about arm's length above the top of the head. Conceptually, the ten soul centers are what many people are usually referring to when describing the nature of each individual chakra.

Almost on a daily basis for about five years, I meditated on, felt, stroked, danced with, made love with these ten centers. Their development seems to be the primary factor in becoming capable of far more conscious communication with my five companions, an ability I did not have when I wrote the first edition of *Sacred Orgasms.* Likewise, the soul center development contributed significantly to the wonderful, wide variety of orgasmic experiences that have unfolded in my life.

None of the ten-center meditations, however, are taught in this *Sacred Orgasms* edition. Instead, my five companions have introduced as an alternative the integration meditations to facilitate a more direct, faster, and smoother path to accomplish what the ten-center meditation has enabled me to experience.

At least, this is my understanding. I do not have five to ten years of personal experience or feedback from others to support these efficacy claims. I must say, however, that a meditation practice that includes daily masturbation or sex with another is likely to be a lot more fun than many other recommendations.

EJACULATION

An additional point of information my companions communicate is that on an ongoing basis, ejaculating is healthier than not ejaculating. Moreover, this applies for both men and women.

My companions' statement, however, runs contrary to a major position in Taoism and some tantric teachings: In ejaculation, men lose energy, and thus ejaculation out through the urethra is best minimized or avoided. Possible alternatives for men are to forego sexual orgasm-ejaculation or to have a retrograde ejaculation, where the ejaculate goes up into the bladder instead of out the penis.

Personally, I sought out and learned some of the Taoist ejaculation retention techniques when, due to some poor health conditions, I started to have major energy drops lasting for two or three days after ejaculation. When I used the techniques, I eliminated much of my energy drop.

Then one day when I had a full, regular ejaculation out the penis (it just felt too good to stop!), I did not have a significant drop in my energy. The only change in my life just prior to this was having all the silver-mercury amalgam fillings removed from my lower teeth. This is an observation, not a recommendation.

So I was quite surprised when my companions said that in general, ejaculation is healthier. My shamanic teacher from Native American traditions, likewise, is a strong advocate of male ejaculation.

Then we also have the companions' statement that women's ejaculation with sexual orgasm is healthier. Until a few decades ago, Western sexology assumed female ejaculation was not even a possibility. Now books and videos advising women on how to ejaculate are common.

I find it amazing that such a simple, natural body function can be such a point of contrasting views. There is no doubt about my companions' position, however. They are quite definite about this teaching.

MY AGREEMENT WITH MY COMPANIONS

One weekend at age twenty-four my life suddenly changed. No significant event occurred. I just realized I had to do something different in my life, and I didn't know what. Within two weeks I had completed my master's thesis and had left the university in the middle of the semester. My first stop was a retreat at a Catholic monastery. A few days later a monk driving into town dropped me off at a freeway entrance to begin my hitchhiking. Getting out of the car, I saw a discarded handwritten sign on the ground. It read, "ANYWHERE."

Looking back, I think of this as the beginning of my spiritual quest. I had no idea, though, I would eventually teach tantric massage, become a sexologist, and that sexuality would be my vehicle on my sacred path.

I especially had no idea I would be in communication with unincarnated beings. It is not at all a role I seek. But what seems to be evolving is the agreement that I will continue receiving knowledge from my companions as long as I am willing to share that knowledge with others.

When I look out into the physical world, I constantly see ethnic cleansing atrocities, racial and religious hatred, and people of one sexual orientation murdering people of another sexual orientation. I see religious and political demagogues and tyrants manipulating hate to their personal advantage. The battle of the sexes, both violent and nonviolent, is a constant. Academically, within the sociological conflict models, this all makes sense.

But deep inside, none of this makes sense to me. I just don't understand humans committing atrocities or authoritarian dominations on such a mass scale. I often feel helpless about changing the world. I often feel rage.

Writing my books has become my primary way of attempting to make a difference. My operating principle is that the ways we as humans relate to our sexuality are often a significant determining factor in how we express ourselves into the world.

I have no absolute certainly that what I am learning from my companions is accurate or effective for others. However, the teachings place sexuality at the center of the sacred circle. This is my truth as well. And what I am learning from my companions is very valuable for me. The orgasms are real!

So I continue with the agreement to teach what I learn from my companions.

I Sex and Orgasm:
Ordinary and
Out-of-the-Ordinary

1. The Spirit and The Flesh

Intercourse and orgasm:
    that's what sex is

Of course, sex is more than intercourse and orgasm
    But this is what most of us think/do/say
        most of our sexual time

There is nothing wrong with
    just intercourse (or any consensual sexual actions)
        and orgasm
    Most of us—not all of us
        would be healthier and happier
        if we did more
        sex
            consensually
            with others and/or ourself
    and orgasm

But there is something terribly *wrong*
    It is not really wrong
    It is a *wrong*
If we have grown up in Western culture
    which is basically Christian culture
    with various threads
    of various philosophies and various theologies
        such as Greek philosophy and Judaism

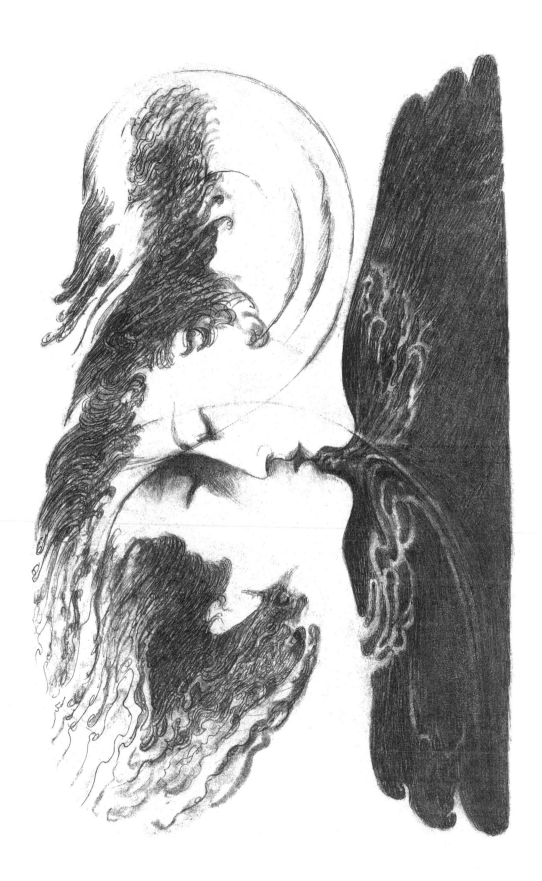

woven in
we have, most of us
in our world view, our cosmology, our psyche
in our core
a basic *wrong*

The *wrong* is *not*
that *spirit* is different than *body*
Concepts allow differentiation
Differentiation can bring us to the wonder
of it all
the incredible, magnificent complexity
of it all

The *wrong*
is that spirit is sacred and
body is profane
The spirit is spiritual, the body is flesh
One is of heaven, the other is of sin

We've got it all wrong

Both are sacred

And orgasm teaches us that

Even if we understand this—that both are sacred,
it may take a lifetime, a long time, a short time
to live it

However, it takes no time to experience it
In orgasm
we go outside of time
we go outside of location
we go outside of identity
outside of mind
we transcend concept, language
In orgasm, there is
no right/wrong
no good/bad
no spiritual/evil

Then after orgasm
we, most of us most of the time,
settle back into the profane

After orgasm
we revel in the orgasm
we savor it
luxuriate in it

classify it
compare it
demean it
depreciate it
hope for it again
try for it again
crave for it again
or just roll over and fall asleep

If we have never had orgasm
        or
if we think we have never had orgasm
        we can fake it
            read about it
            hope for it
            be afraid of it
            ache for it
                    and not know why we ache
            work on it

Sacred Orgasms, the book, is not about
                    mature orgasms
                    or multiple orgasms
        it is not about how not to *lose* an erection
            how not to ejaculate too soon
            how not to ejaculate with an orgasm
                    (for those who can and don't want to)
            how to ejaculate
                    (for those who can't and want to)

Sacred Orgasms is about shifting the paradigm
        about stepping outside our framework
        about stepping into a different reality
The paradigm in *Sacred Orgasms*
        holds both the spirit and the body
                as sacred
        Likewise, both are profane
                if we choose to live our life that way

Religious teachings
        most of them most of the time
        hold the spirit as sacred and
                the flesh as profane
        Though through the ages
                mysticism has sometimes
                        expressed reverence
                for the marriage of the body and the soul
                occurring during the ecstatic experience

Scientific teachings,
     having themselves attained a religious fervor
          most of the time,
     hold matter as profane
     Thus, the body is profane
          (though miraculous)
     The spirit, if measurable,
          would be profane
          as well

Sexology
     is the interdisciplinary study of sexuality
          especially human sexuality
     Being principally scientific, this field of study
          views the body as profane
               most of the time:
          how often we do it
             intercourse, other sex actions, orgasm
               with whom
               with what
               when
          how to do it
          how not to do it
          how to do it better
     From sexology,
          an immense amount of information
          and a valuable set of therapeutic procedures
          are bringing us—some of us
          out of a millennium or two of
             sexual suppression
             sexual repression
             sexual oppression
          slowly, awkwardly sometimes
             Probably there is no other way out

There is another -ology
     Named after Eros,
          the ancient Greek god of love
          (later called Cupid by the Romans),
erotology
     is the study of sexual pleasure,
          of lovemaking rituals
     It is the study of the representations of our sexual nature
          in sculpture, in paintings, in music,
          in film, in literature
     This -ology, unfortunately, is more of a coined term
          than an extensive field of study
     Here, usually, there is a reverence
          for the body
          for the senses

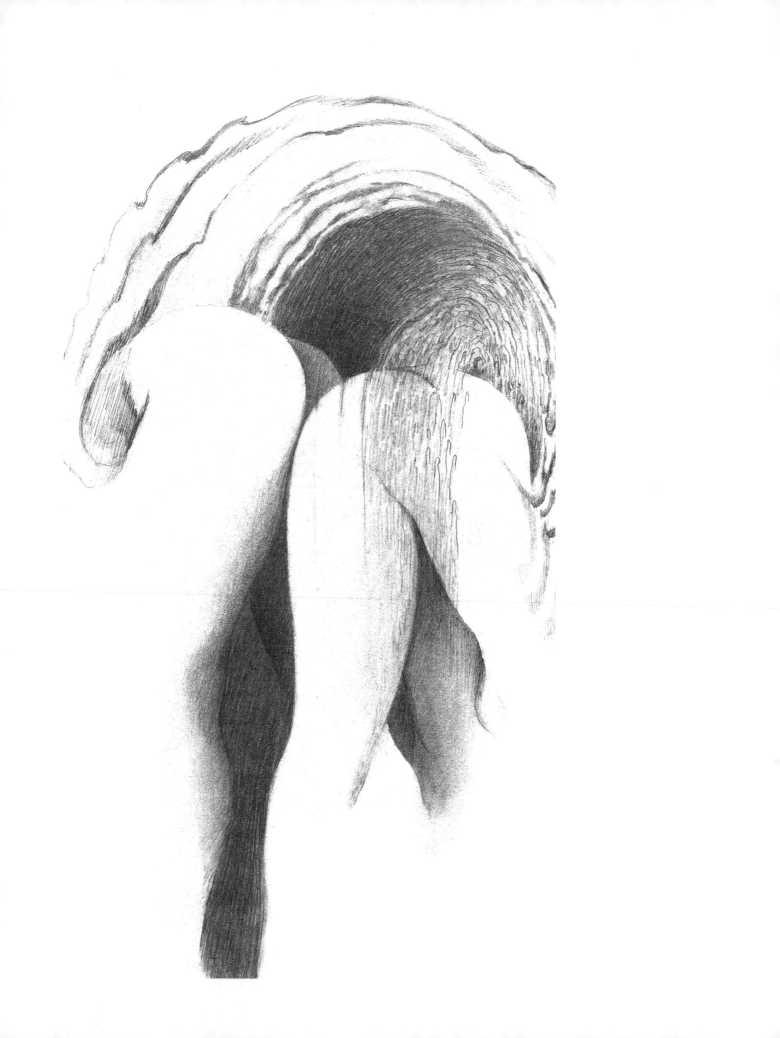

a recognition of love
Spirit is affirmed, some of the time,
though the emphasis is physical

Contemporary sexuality, however,
is more what it is
more,
probably,
because of the artist
Artists, many of them much of the time,
are outside
outside of the mainstream
outside of the power structures
outside of the cultural embargoes
the dancer, the musician, the singer,
the actor/actress express
the sculptor, the painter, the filmmaker reveal
the poet, the songwriter, the writer remind us of
our soul
our beauty
our passion
our joy
our love
our wonder
Artists
far more than the high priest/esses
of religion and of science
have liberated
celebrated
proclaimed
consecrated
the spirit and the body

When we interweave these institutions
with a myriad of other patterns
we have *contemporary sex, ordinary sex*
which for most of us ordinarily
looks like this:
Subject:
one person
or two people physically together
female/male, male/male, female/female
or possibly more than two
Verb:
to have sexual actions
usually with the genitals
often with the mouth and/or hands
usually on one or more of these:
clitoris, head of penis,
G spot, prostate gland,
perhaps other places

Object:

       orgasm

           hoping for multiple orgasms

           hoping for simultaneous orgasms

Adverbs and Adjectives

       —such as *gentle, tenderly, passionately:*

           this is the language

           of lovemaking and romance

There can be many variations to these patterns

It's simply a matter of choice

       and there are lots of choices

2. Out-of-the-Ordinary Orgasms

Sexual orgasm

       in contemporary Western sexology

       and for most of us personally most of the time

basically is

       muscular tension release

       (Definitely, though,

           not all tension releases

           are orgasms)

This is the pattern:

       A build up of muscular tension (myotonia)

           and tumescence (vasocongestion,

               engorgement of blood)

           often with body movements accompanying

       An orgasm may follow:

           a series of involuntary muscular contractions

           in the pelvic floor

           producing

               in the male, often though not always

                   an ejaculation of fluid

                   out through the urethra

               in the female, sometimes

                   but not for most most of the time

                   an ejaculation of fluid

                   out through the urethra

       Finally, a general release of muscular tension occurs

Multiple orgasms basically means that

       instead of a more-or-less complete release

           of muscular tension

       another cycle begins with tension buildup

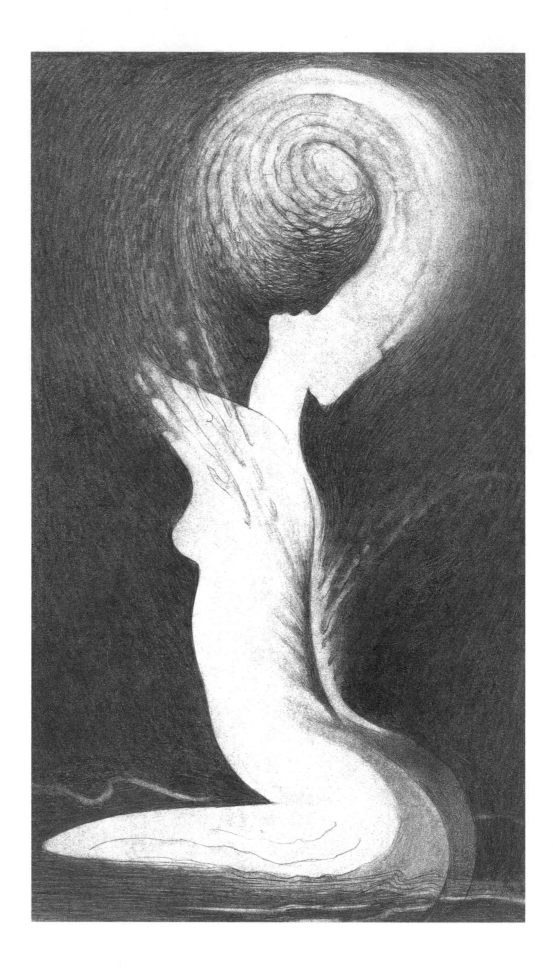

followed by involuntary pelvic-floor contractions
followed by a general release of muscular tension
This can continue for a period of time
with an ejaculation during none, some, or all
of the series of pelvic-floor contractions

There is, of course, more to orgasm than physiological phases:
feelings
emotions
intense experiences
an altered state of consciousness
Our model of orgasm, however,
is as what science defines/describes:
basically, physical tension release

It is a valuable model, a useful model
Orgasm as a series of physiological changes
is an excellent way to frame / think of
what many of us experience most of the time
when we have sex
with others, with ourself
It's the some-of-the-other times
the some-of-the-other experiences
the some-of-the-other orgasms
the mystical ones
that aren't explained by / understood from
a physiological definition

Sometimes, even if there is a
tension/contractions/release cycle,
this is only incidental to the totality
of the experience
Or
the context is nonsexual and/or
the activity is nonsexual
Or
something about the experience
does not
look/smell/taste/feel/sound like
the textbook definitions of sex and orgasm

Some of these experiences are once-in-a-lifetime occurrences
—a sort of cosmic orgasm choosing us
Some have been consciously repeated
Some have been consciously attempted
often to remain only attempted

The list of *out-of-the-ordinary orgasms*,
a term for a diverse spectrum of experiences,
is long

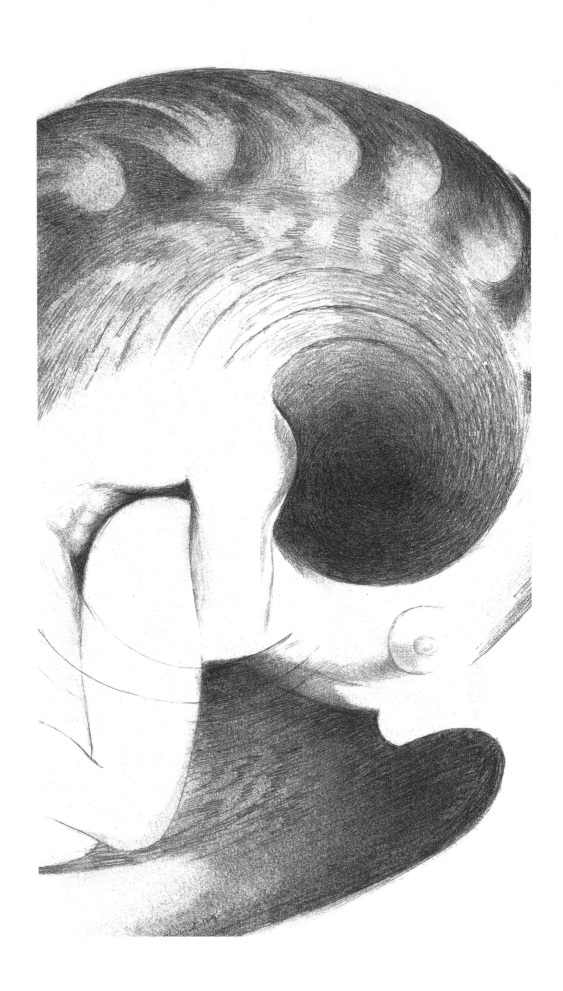

Here are only a few
     without genital stimulation that I have
     experienced, heard about, and/or read about
       (though out-of-the-ordinary orgasms
        can definitely occur
        with genital stimulation as well):

while listening to *Tristan and Isolde*
    by Wagner

while smelling a night-blooming jasmine

while climbing a rope

while taking the first bite of a peach

while receiving a massage
    between the toes
    on the thighs
    on the abdomen
    around the ears
    on the left triceps muscle
    on the back of the neck

while giving a massage
    on the back of the neck

while doing breathing exercises

while only fantasizing

while watching someone teach, fully clothed,
    how to do meditative sex

while meditating quietly

while videotaping a space shuttle blast off
    when the rumble of the bass sound waves hit

while watching waves crashing on the rocks
    for half an hour

while skydiving, immediately after jumping out of a plane
    for the first time

while watching dolphins
    swimming/leaping in the water

while embracing nonsexually

while lying beside someone chanting

while running the shower on shoulder muscles

while reading the manuscript of this book

while touching the wetness of a tomato plant

while riding on buses, on subways
    feeling the vibrations in the pelvis

while hugging a tree

while lying on a large rock
    just feeling the energy of the rock

while having a chiropractic adjustment
    in the lower back

Once a friend bluntly explained that
    St. Teresa of Avila's ecstatic, mystical communions
        with God
      really were orgasms
    (St. Teresa was a sixteenth-century nun
      who, during the Spanish Inquisition,
      wrote about her spiritual life)
    "Sex with God," I thought
      "What a way to keep celibacy vows!"

Another friend tells of making love with his partner
    Both are suddenly looking down
      at a couple below, on a blanket on the grass
        just like themselves
    Then they realize
      it is themselves
        they later report to each other

Others tell of dreams
    vivid dreams
    where they are having orgasms
        in the dream *and* in their physical body
    In the dream they are making love
      with their partner
      with someone they do not know
      with energies without definite form
      with water flowing around their pelvis and
        through their legs
In one vivid dream a person is being led toward *The Light*,
    a massive, continuous, orgasmic explosion

While watching television, a friend's pelvis
            began to move, until he had an orgasm
      Looking around at the rest of his family
            he realized no one else
                  had had the same experience
                  from the TV
      He was only two years old

Several friends have exclaimed
      they have experienced orgasms
            while giving birth
            while breast feeding

Religious services are not excluded:
It was a hot, humid Sunday morning church service
      with hand-held fans barely lifting the air
      when I saw a congregation member *get happy*
            as it is sometimes called
This was no somber religious gathering
The preacher, as the high priest/ess is termed there,
      was giving a sermon building in fervor
      while various members of the congregation
            responded vocally
            in rhythm
            to the preacher's invocation
                  of the Holy Spirit
                  as well as the human spirit
The whole church broke out in hymn
      hands clapping
      the organ and the piano pounding a primordial beat
      voices lifted in praise
As the religious passions escalated
      one of the several congregation members
            dressed in all-white in the front pew
      became even more expressive than the others
Her arms and torso movement appeared to become uncontrollable
      her singing converted to moaning screams
As a novice to such gatherings, I had been forewarned
      by my friend who nodded to me
      that the woman was OK
      as she collapsed to the floor
            her body vibrating and proclaiming itself
Several of her all-white-clad companions swiftly moved
      over to her assistance and fanned her
After a while, while others continued singing,
      she was raised back to her seat in the pew
She was more than OK—she had *gotten happy*
      She was in spiritual ecstasy

A few years later I reflected
            somewhat seriously, somewhat jokingly
      getting happy is an orgasm
            intense, expressive, communal
            with the Holy Spirit perhaps
            with herself
            I don't know
      but still an orgasm

Another few years later
      while reading the Kinsey report
            on sexual behavior in the human male
      I read basically the same description of orgasm
            as *getting happy*
      It, however, was not about
            church service experiences
            It was a description
            of orgasms in infants

Another friend reminisces of her spiritual master in India
      He would sit in meditation
            with a small gathering of followers
      After a while, their bodies would
            vibrate, undulate, shake . . .
            eventually slump/jump/writhe/swoon
                  to the floor in bliss
            only to be carried away by attendants
      so that the next soon-to-be-orgasmic group
            could be escorted in
      There was no sex, as most of us would call it
      The spiritual teacher was
            making love with energy
            without touching an erogenous zone

Whenever there is a paradigm shift
      there is a turning point
            a catalytic event
      when the cognitive dissonance is too dissonant
            and we let go of the reigning
                  concepts, definitions, framework
      If we believe the world is flat
            but we have just sailed west continuously
                  and have returned to our starting point
                  without falling off the world
            we might change
                  our concept that the world is flat
      Here is my turning point:

It was late one evening while I was working in my office
Feeling that something was different
        that there had been an energy change
        I sat down in meditation
First I sensed the *presence* of a new friend
        We had met on a business phone call a month earlier
            and though we had never been face-to-face,
            several phone conversations had established
                a beginning friendship
        Even if it were not my friend
            I felt I could trust the presence
        and so relaxed into the energies near me
Within about a few seconds
        my breathing expanded
            in sigh-like movements
A gentle but definite
        flow of energy lifted up from my head
        to a foot or two above me
Then everything was calm
Though I had had
        no sexual feelings, no erection, no ejaculation
        I suddenly thought, "She just had an orgasm."
It was late in the evening
        even later three thousand miles east
            at my friend's home
        but she had said it was OK to phone late
My first words: "Did you just have an orgasm?"
She burst out laughing as she said, "Yes."
        (The phone call was not an interruption
            as she was alone)
My friend has more psychic abilities
        than most people I know
        but to send/project/present her energy
        three thousand miles away . . .

This had *not* been a mystical dream
            a theoretical fantasy
            a delusion of ecstasy
        The exact person, the exact time, the exact event
        All totally verified

More was to come
In the following months
        simultaneous orgasms
            with my long-distance friend began to occur
                simultaneous three thousand miles apart
In the middle of the night
        sleeping alone and apart from each other
        when we awoke in orgasm
            we would check our clocks

In a morning phone call
      the orgasm times were verified as the same
            with adjustments for time zone differences
Intensely "pleasurable sexual orgasms"
      was her description
For me: an electric-shock-like sensation
      throughout my energy field
            with my physical body whipping across the bed
Pleasurable, nonsexual, no erection, no ejaculation
      but *orgasm* is the only word I would use
While this was the turning point,
      the long-distance orgasms
            turned out to be only the beginning
            of my journey to a new paradigm

It was a hot summer evening
            even hotter because the windows were closed
            so as not to awaken the neighbors again
as a friend / lover / meditation partner and I
      were having good ole contemporary sex
            the coital kind, of a safer-sex, condom-sex variety
                though not in the missionary position
We had begun with quiet meditation
            back to back, breathing in unison
      then some massage and caressing
Somewhere along the way
            our bodies flowed into intercourse
      There was no rush,
            though, indeed, there was
                sweat and passion
At some point my orgasm began
            with the usual
                pelvic-floor contractions and
                ejaculation
            as my partner went into her orgasm
                which in her usual fashion
                was long and intense
Shortly my own orgasm completed
Then, unanticipated, a few seconds later,
            as her long orgasm continued,
         my back and neck began to arch
         with my mouth stretching open
         and the sounds of orgasm erupting again
            through my chest and throat
                joining my partner's screams

Everything was just like
            my orgasm of a few moments earlier—except
            there were

no pelvic-floor contractions
no ejaculation
This was an orgasm that felt just like a sexual orgasm
in every way and everywhere
except in my pelvis
It was as if my partner's core
was pulling me up into her explosion
up into one, encompassing, merged,
energetic orgasm
One thing for certain though,
even the closed windows
did not keep the neighborhood quiet that night

Neither this energetic orgasm
nor the earlier long-distance simultaneous orgasms
were to be anything like an experience a year later
I was visiting a desert area
noted for its power spots, or energy vortexes
This is a place where Native Americans came
for ceremony
where stone cathedral formations
spire toward the heavens
where boulders aeons ago came to rest on buttes
giving them the appearance of
birds, lizards, other animals,
and mythical beings
It is called *sacred earth* there
and so a Catholic chapel had been constructed
framed around a magnificent, tall cross
facing the south
But the sacred earth was to be found, for me,
outside
several yards to the east
and here it was I came to meditate on several afternoons
Each time, to find the place
for that afternoon's meditation
I would from inside myself
feel the earth
This time I selected the middle of three tiers
where ancient waters
had carved Rubenesque beauty
into the red-toned stone
Sitting down
with my legs dangling over a ledge
I closed my eyes
and began my usual inner observation
of sensations
in and around my body
Almost immediately my back began to arch
I had felt energy in this desert area before

but this time it was particularly intense
and so I leaned back
allowing the warm stone to cradle me
There, before I could even become surprised,
a blast of light and sound surged into my head
blinding my senses
for only a moment maybe, I am not certain
Maybe it was like the light that blinded Paul
as he journeyed through the desert
toward Damascus
All I remember next
was a sound inside my head,
a sound which seemed to be
the humming roar of the light
in the center of my brain
There was no up or down
as I came back to consciousness
only the movement of my legs dangling
and my hands
searching for gravity
bracing the stone

I had felt a surge not unlike a sexual orgasm
except that the explosion was in my head
somewhere in the center of my consciousness
Though there were
no sexual feelings, no erection, no ejaculation
again, the experience was pleasurable
again, my best description is *orgasm*

While these experiences
with my long-distance friend
the energetic orgasm following the sexual orgasm
and the Earthgasm
were not consciously attempted or sought after
they did not occur in a vacuum
There had been many years of conscious *seeking*
There had to be more meaning to existence
than what I had felt/seen/heard/learned
in church and in school

Many teachers and many teachings
from other traditions and
from outside mainstream culture
have been sought / discovered / bumped into
along my path
Without these teachers and teachings
there would not have been a paradigm shift, probably

The descriptions, the interpretations
       of the four paths
           that follow
    are mine
These are my
       overgeneralizations
       oversimplifications
       often personal reinterpretations
           of teachings
           I have read, heard, and/or experienced
What makes these teachings from the four paths different
       than mainstream thinking
           is that *spiritual* and *sexual* are not in opposition
       The spirit and the body
           are integral parts of wholeness
       where *at-one-ment* rather than *atonement*
              is central

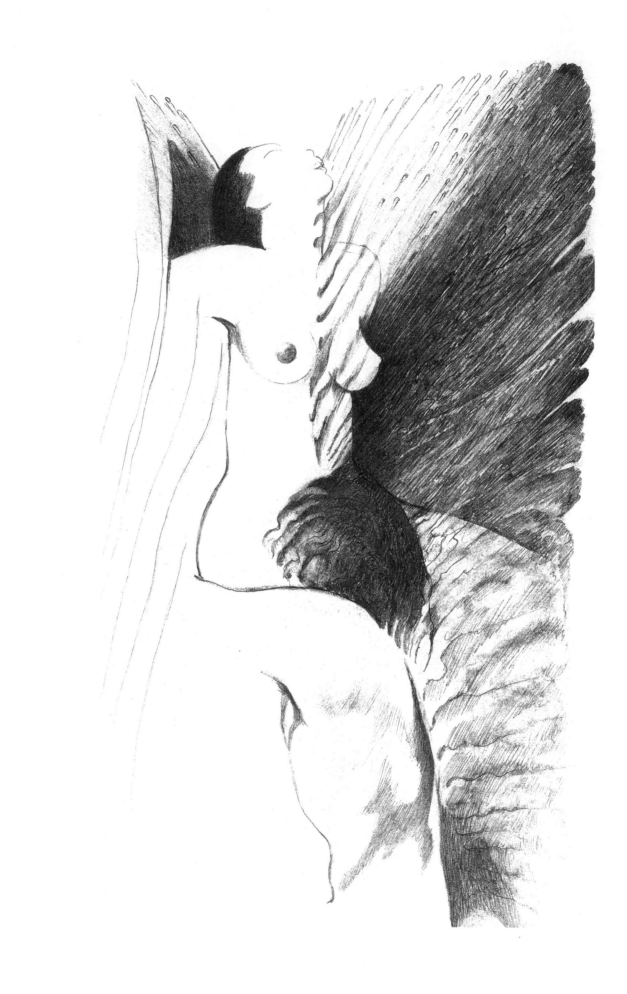

II Four Paths

3. Tantra

Tantra (pronounced *tahn´ trah*)
> today in the Western world
> has come to mean
> *spiritual sexuality*
> > Indeed, *tantra* has almost become
> > the generic term
> > > for all styles/traditions of
> > > > spiritual/meditative sexuality

Tantra
> which is part of both
> > some Hindu and some Buddhist teachings
> actually is far more encompassing
> > than *sex done spiritually*

Tantra embraces all:
> birth, death, pleasure, pain
> wealth, poverty, beauty, ugliness
> joy, sadness, anger, fear, ecstasy
> sex, celibacy

Tantra basically is a teaching of acceptance
> > a teaching of nonattachment
> When we are *grasping* an object/action/outcome
> > we are attached
> > there is no freedom
> When we are *avoiding* an object/action/outcome

we are attached
there is no freedom
It is through the acceptance of all
as it is
that we become/are free
Acceptance
is not submission
is not giving up
Here, acceptance means nonattachment

By embracing the present
while letting go of
expectations of the future and
comparisons with the past
we can fully dance with life
(and death)
There is no good/bad
no right/wrong
no spiritual/evil
only suffering
unless/until we let go of our attachments

Neither being sexual nor being celibate
is preferable
If we feel superior/inferior because we are/aren't sexual,
we are attached
If we feel superior/inferior because
we are/aren't celibate,
we are attached
If we feel superior/inferior when we do/don't masturbate,
we are attached
If we feel superior/inferior because we do/don't do
heterosexual actions
or homosexual actions
or bisexual actions
we are attached
If we feel superior/inferior because we do/don't
go to church/synagogue/the ashram/etc.
pray/meditate
tithe/donate
or do any other
religiously sanctioned action
we are attached
There are other words for superior:
pious, proud, arrogant, egotistic, patronizing,
condescending
There are other words for inferior:
guilt, shame, worthless, incompetent, unimportant
dumb, awkward
It is neither in the doing-ness nor in the non-doing-ness

It is in how we relate to an object/action/outcome
      that makes the difference
If we are attached to an object/action/outcome,
      sooner or later we will be in
          physical/emotional pain/discomfort
      when the object is no longer there
          or is there when we don't want it there
      when the action is too slow, too fast, too . . .
      when the outcome is different than
          we had hoped/expected
sooner or later we will be in
          what the Buddha termed *dukkha*
            (pronounced *doo´ kah*)
          which is loosely translated as suffering

So, do we simply
      stop doing the bad behaviors?
      start doing the good behaviors?

The answer is not in the stopping or starting
      Rather, we shift how we relate
          to what we are/do/have
      We transform the grasping energy
      We transform the avoiding energy

How to transform energy?
      To find that answer, those answers
      Is why some of us search the world
          for gurus
             or any other form of high priest/ess
      That is why some of us spend years
          sitting at a master's feet
      That is why some of us enter monasteries and convents

When we are able to
      transform/convert/transubstantiate/transmute the energy
          at will
      we are liberated
      we are enlightened
      we are in nirvana
      or in Christian terms
          we have entered
          the Kingdom of God / Queendom of Goddess

There are many paths
      to learn ways to transform energy
Sex is one of those paths

Sex is a path to liberation
Sex is a path to enlightenment
Sex is a path to the King/Queendom of God/dess

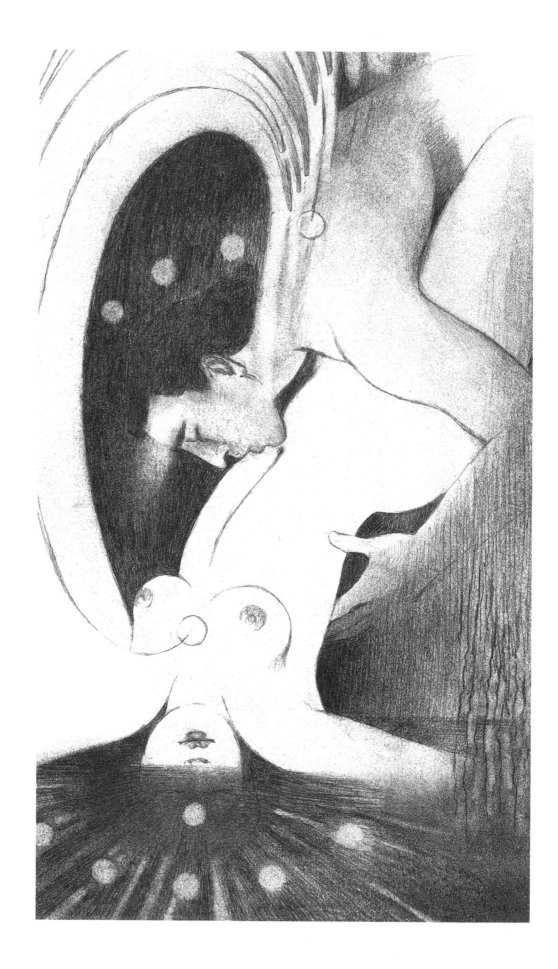

Here, though,
  sex is usually not the sex
    that most of us do most of the time
  Here, sex is not
    just the contemporary sex characterized earlier
A more accurate concept for sex
  intended to transform energy
    would be *meditative sex*
  Some would say *spiritual sex, sacred sex*
  Either term is suitable
    as long as we do not slip into a belief
      that spiritual sex is superior to
        flesh sex
        base sex
        friction sex
        passionate sex
        raw sex

Meditative sex has its varied forms
Contemporary sex has its varied forms
  Sometimes the forms look the same
    Sometimes the forms look very different

In many schools of tantra
  there are at least four major types of meditative forms:
    mantra (*mon´ trah*)
    mudra (*moo´ drah*) and asana (*ah´ sah nah*)
    pranayama (*prah nah yah´ mah*)
    yantra (*yawn´ trah*)

A mantra is a sound or series of sounds
      sometimes vocally produced
      sometimes silently imagined
      sometimes sounds from nature,
          from musical instruments,
        or other sources
  OM is the most noted
  Amen is similar in the West
  Likewise, The Lord's Prayer is a mantra
  Ummmm and *oooh* could be sexual mantras

A mudra is a body gesture or posture
      especially with the hands
An asana is specifically a body posture
    In meditations, gestures and postures
        are often combined
      Jesus is often depicted standing
        with his arms, hands, and fingers
        in definite positions
      The palms placed together while praying
        is another mudra

The Buddha sitting cross-legged is common
in the East
Sexual positions can be asanas

Pranayama is conscious breathing in specific patterns
Rapid inhalation and exhalation
through the nostrils
is one of the more well-known
Eastern forms
Sports training and singing training
often utilize certain breathing techniques
Sometimes Western sex therapy teaches
that holding our breath
inhibits the orgasm response—so breathe!

A yantra is a visual representation
often using geometric shapes
A yantra can be observed externally
or visualized internally
A mandala is a yantra with a circular motif
Symbols, colors, pictures, all can be yantras
The cross,
with the horizontal bar
at different positions,
is common across cultures
and across the ages
Botticelli's *Birth of Venus* is a renaissance yantra

Meditation, often,
simply
is doing a mantra, mudra/asana, pranayama,
and/or yantra
At least, this is what meditation looks like
These are the forms we often learn first

Actually,
meditation is the conscious
awareness/attentiveness/mindfulness
while we are doing the meditation forms

Actually,
meditation is the conscious
awareness/attentiveness/mindfulness
during every moment
regardless of the form/nonform
we are doing / not doing
if we remain consciously aware

So what is meditative sex?

Here is one image, using tantric forms:
> sitting cross-legged in coitus
>> with our sexual partner
> while chanting OM
> while gazing into our partner's left eye

It's that simple
> —unless we have difficulty sitting cross-legged

While this is accurate,
> it is only the humorous answer

Compared to contemporary sex,
> tantric sex is far more ceremonial
> There are elaborate methods of
>> nurturing and stimulating the senses
>> expressing devotion
>> honoring the sacredness of sexual union
> Such a tantric sex ritual,
>> sometimes known as *maithuna*
>>> (pronounced *my thu´nah*),
>> is at the other end of the spectrum
>>> than the *quickie*
>> Though, in tantric philosophy,
>>> both would be sacred
>> Maithuna is more intricate
>>> in time, intent, and activity

The forms, however, are not what make
> meditative sex meditative
It is the approach:
> the awareness
> the attentiveness
> the mindfulness
These make sex meditative
Being in the present
> being aware of sensations of skin touching skin
> tuning into the pressure building in our pelvis
>> or elsewhere
> hearing the sound of our breath,
>> our partner's breath
>>> if we are with another/others
> feeling our heart beat
> being mindful of the muscular tension building
All these
> without the past or the future
> And if our mind goes to the past, to the future
>> we are even aware *also*
>>> of the past/future images/thoughts
All this is meditative sex
> regardless of the forms

regardless of whether we are doing what we term
masturbation, oral sex, anal sex,
genital-genital sex, tantric sex rituals,
or any other form of consensual sex

Some of us have been doing meditative sex all along
at least to some degree
at least some of the time

But to understand meditative sex
is to understand part of the paradigm shift:
we are more
than a physical body
Not *more* in the sense of
mental, emotional, physical, spiritual aspects
Rather, *more* in the sense
that the physical body is only *one*
of several systems

Tantric teachings hold that
there are other
coexisting, interacting systems
that each of us has
in varying degrees of development

Systems is my term
Some other terms are
energies
energy fields
subtle bodies
energy bodies
light bodies

These other systems are *subtle*
in the sense that
the effects in the physical, material world
are not obvious
to most of us
most of the time

The most commonly taught subtle energy system is
the *chakras*
(pronounced *shah´ kras*)
This is a system of energy centers
often thought of as along an imaginary axis
in the core of our physical body
from the bottom of our pelvis
(commonly called the *first chakra*)
to the inside top of our head
(commonly called the *seventh chakra*)

Most schools of meditation teach that
          there are seven principal chakras
              along the imaginary axis
       with secondary chakras
           throughout the body,
           the number varying in different traditions

A clarification of our language:
      chakras are not *in* the physical body
          though a chakra's *location*
             can be conveniently identified
      by naming an area of our physical body

Chakras, in Sanskrit,
          means *wheels* or *discs*
     they have also been described as
          cone-shaped vortexes

More important, though, is their function:
      Chakras are often considered
          energy transformers
      Analogously to the physical body's
          digestion process transforming food,
      the chakras transform energies
          for us to utilize

Tantric meditations in general, usually, are designed
          to awaken
          to develop
          to utilize
     the energies and the functions
     of the chakras and other subtle energy systems
Likewise, tantric sex rituals,
          and most other forms of meditative sex,
     are designed to do the same:
          to awaken
          to develop
          to utilize
     the energies and the functions
     of the chakras and other subtle energy systems
The conscious
          awareness/attentiveness/mindfulness
          is, in a sense,
          the key to the doors
             of these not-so-physical systems
             as well as the physical body system

Herein lies a fundamental contrast
     to the Western
          spirit-higher-than-the-flesh framework:

There is no denial of the physical body
>> no subjugation
>> no demeaning morality
Similarly, the physical body is
>> neither idealized, glorified, nor idolized

4. Taoism

T'ai Chi Ch'uan (pronounced *tie gee chowan*)
>> is an ancient martial art
>>> with roots in Taoism,
>>> an ancient spiritual philosophy
>>>> from China
>> (Tao is pronounced *dow*)

When we observe the ritual,
>> we see a slow-motion dance
>>> of flowing agility and keen balance

Once a master was in the middle
>> of the t'ai chi ch'uan ritual
>> A passing sparrow lighted on the swaying branch
>>> unaware
>>>> it was a floating hand
>>>>> of the master
>>>>>> effortlessly balanced upon the Earth
After resting,
>> the sparrow was ready to continue flight
>> To gain the necessary momentum to begin flight
>>> the sparrow thrust off with its legs
However, the master
>>> being very sensitive
>> yielded to the force,
>>> the hand descending
>>> the exact distance, direction, and velocity
>>> of the thrust
Without a resisting surface,
>> the sparrow could not take flight

Recognizing the bird's desire to depart
>> the master chose to steady the hand
>>> offering the necessary resistance
>>> for the sparrow's thrust
>>>> to flight
This is a story about
balance and yielding
>> which are central in Taoism

Balance can be
>between Heaven, Human Being, and Earth
>between yin and yang
>>(pronounced *yen* and *yahng*)
>>which could be translated as
>>>receptive and active, respectively
>balanced in the flow of energy
>>through the acupuncture meridians
>balanced between the Five Elements
>>in traditional Chinese medicine:
>>>fire, water, wood, metal, earth
>In Western concepts,
>>there would be a balance
>>between the mental, emotional, physical, spiritual

Yielding
>is characterized by the Chinese term *wu wei*
>>(pronounced *woo way*):
>allowing things to flow in accordance
>>with the nature of things
>Wu wei is noticeably similar
>>to the nongrasping and nonavoidance
>>of tantric philosophy
When we are in the river of life
>we can struggle paddling upstream
>we can hurry paddling downstream
>or we can *allow* the river
>>to carry us at its own pace
>>while we enjoy the scenery
>>>along the way

In our quest for sex and orgasm,
>contemporary sex would look very different
>if we were to incorporate
>>Taoist balance and yielding
>Sex, probably, would be
>>less goal oriented
>>less of a performance
>Sex, probably, would be
>>slower
>>longer
>>more exploratory
>>more sensual
>>more intimate

Health and longevity
>also are central in Taoist thought
For us, as human beings,
>the extent to which
>>we have health and longevity

depends, greatly, on the extent to which
we live in harmony
with the changing seasons
with social, political, and cultural changes
with the cycles in the bodily functions
with all change,
which is basic to existence

To live in harmony with changes,
Taoism offers practical teachings:
how to make wise decisions
how to balance our diet
which herbs to use and
which acupuncture/acupressure points
to stimulate/sedate
to maintain and restore health
which meditations to strengthen
our internal organs and glands
how to use sex and sexual energy
to improve health,
to harmonize relationships,
and to increase spiritual realization

A Taoist teaching about The Seven Glands
helps us to understand
how sex and sexual energy
are part of health and longevity
The seven glands in one of the classic texts are the
pineal gland
pituitary gland
thyroid gland
thymus
pancreas
adrenal glands, and
the sex glands, here defined as
in the male: the prostate and the testes
in the female: the ovaries, uterus, vagina,
and breasts

In The Seven Glands teaching,
which is more analogous
than scientific,
each gland is dependent (at least indirectly) on the others
for its energy
If a gland is excessively drained of its vitality,
such as in an illness,
all the other glands are drained
If a gland has extra energy,
all the other glands benefit

To increase the energy level
            of the glandular system
        there are various methods
One specifically for the sex glands
            is translated as The Deer Exercise
        Basically, this is
            the contraction (and later the relaxation)
            of the pelvic floor muscles
        In the tantric tradition, a similar method
                is called the mula bandha
                (pronounced *moo lah bahn´ dah*)
        In the West, a similar method
                is called Kegel Exercises,
                or simply, Kegels,
                (pronounced *Kay´gulls*)
                named after a physician
                who re-*invented* similar exercises

For many of us,
        sexual intercourse is
            a way to feel pleasure
            a way to express love
In Taoist teachings,
        sexual intercourse can also be
        a healing method
To understand coitus as a healing,
        it helps to understand the theory of reflexology
        In the West, foot reflexology already
            is a common massage form
        Here, different parts of the body
                correspond to different parts of the foot
            By massaging or applying pressure
                    on a place on the foot,
                we can have a healing effect
                    on another part of the body
        For example, massaging certain places
            on the big toe
            can eliminate/reduce a headache,
                according to the theory
                and many peoples' experience
In Taoist teachings,
            there is also a reflexology of the genitals
        By having sexual intercourse in specific ways/positions,
            certain organs are affected
            such that a healing effect occurs
        (See Diagram 1 for the organ systems on the genitals)
Personally, I know of no testimonials
        supporting or refuting this healing theory
            developed in ancient times
        But it does sound like a wonderful way
            to play doctor

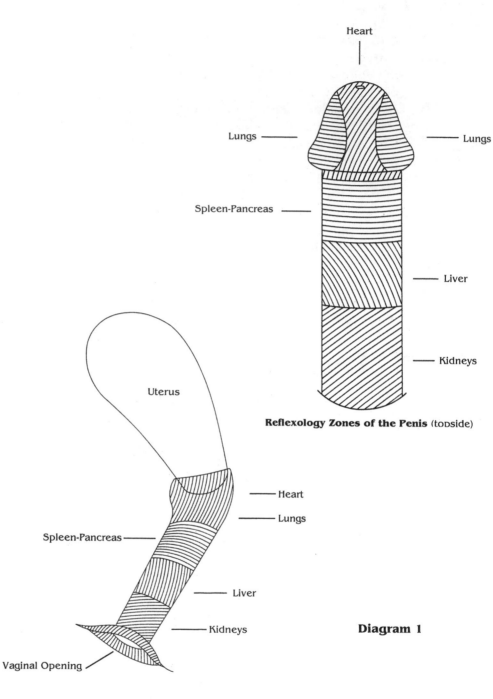

Heart

Lungs ——— ——— Lungs

Spleen-Pancreas ———

——— Liver

——— Kidneys

Reflexology Zones of the Penis (topside)

Uterus

——— Heart

——— Lungs

Spleen-Pancreas ———

——— Liver

——— Kidneys

Vaginal Opening ———

Diagram 1

Reflexology Zones of the Vagina

5. Quodoushka

Many of us
        who have felt/sensed/known/hoped
        that sexuality is not in opposition
                to spirituality
        have turned to the East
                to India, China, Tibet, Japan
        for new teachings, different approaches

But such teachings were already here
        in North America
                though Native Americans had learned
                        for their own survival
                not to talk about such teachings
                in the presence
                        of oppressive armies
                        with oppressive moralities

Quodoushka
        (pronounced *kwah doesh´ ka*)
        could be translated as
                spiritual sexuality
        Some of the practices and concepts have
                similarities with tantric and Taoist sexuality

In the Quodoushka tradition
        children were taught from a young age
                about the beauty of sexuality
                about having reverence for sexual union
                about honoring those with whom
                        we express our sexuality
At puberty, after the rites of passage
                into adulthood,
        the young adult would study
                for several years
        with a *fireperson*
                the gender of whom depended on
                the young adult's sexual orientation
A fireperson is a medicine man/woman
                (a high priest/ess)
        specializing in *fire-medicine*,
                the ancient knowledge of spiritual sexuality
        Their teachings included
                what most of us would call
                the physical art of lovemaking
                        one-to-one with the young adult
                (The recently *discovered* G spot, for example,
                        has been known for centuries
                as *The Secret Fire-Trigger of the Serpent*)

Another major Quodoushka teaching was
how our sexual partner(s) are a mirror
of the different aspects of ourselves,
not at all unlike some of the current
Western psychological theories
However, very unlike what most of us
were ever taught
in school or in church/synagogue,
the young adult learned about
the chakras and other subtle energy systems
—directly, experientially
sometimes in vision quests
sometimes in sexual union
with another
In the Quodoushka tradition,
the subtle energy systems
are not just esoteric/hidden/secret teachings
solely for the medicine person
Development of the chakras, the aura, the shields,
the luminous sphere
and other translated terms for subtle energies
was a standard part of education

In contrast to contemporary Western education,
many Native American traditions teach
the sacredness of all existence
Before I was introduced
to even the basics of Quodoushka teachings,
the shaman
(another word for medicine person,
high priest/ess)
began with the Sacred Pipe Ceremony
After the stem and bowl were joined
and the herbal mixture lit,
soon began
the invocation to the Great Spirit, Wakantanka
the invocation to Grandfather Sun
and Grandmother Earth
then the invocations to the
powers/energies/essences/beauty
of the Four Directions
South
West
North
East
of the Four Worlds
the sacred minerals
the Sands
the Rocks/Stones
the Gems

                    the Crystals
                    the Mixed Ores and Metals
          the sacred plants
                    the Grasses and Grains
                    the Herbs and Shrubs
                    the Fruits and Flowers
                    the Trees
                    the Teacher Plants
          the sacred animals
                    the Swimmers
                    the Creepers and Crawlers
                    the Four Leggeds
                    the Winged Ones
                    the Two Leggeds
                              and Mythical Animals
          the sacred humans
                    the Red
                    the Black
                    the White
                    the Yellow
                    the Mixed
     of the sacred ancestor spirits

     In Biblical terms, the Sacred Pipe Ceremony said,
          "Be still and know that I am God"
     My translation:
          "Be aware and experience the sacred presence"

Only after this psychological/spiritual platform
          was laid
     did the sensual and sexual instruction begin
Even the basic teaching tool
     is a sacred symbol:
               the wheel / the circle / the sacred hoop

On the wheel
     the positions are represented by the cardinal directions:
          North, East, South, West
     and the noncardinals:
          Northeast, Southeast, Southwest, Northwest
Each of these positions has
          certain qualities/characteristics/meanings
     Almost any topic (it seems)
          such as sexuality, the seasons,
               colors, relationships
     can be examined/taught/appreciated
     from the diverse aspects of the positions
          around the wheel
The wheel,
          unlike most scientific linear thought,

has no *beginning*, no *end*
There are no superior places, no inferior places
            just different places, different viewing points
            each with its value and meaning
A different position is a different experience
            in which we can participate
            if we choose

There is a wheel for different types of lovers:
            in the North: the Career/Goal-Oriented Lover
            in the East: the Temple Priest/ess Lover
            in the South: the Shy, Curious Lover
            in the Southwest: the Explorer/Adventurer Lover
            in the West: the Wanton/Lusty Lover
                        and so on
Most of us, most of the time
            are *stuck* in one of these positions on the wheel
                        we are unimaginative
                        we are reluctant to leave our comfort zone
                        we are socially conditioned as to what
                                    the different genders *should* do,
                                    the different roles we *should* play
The Quodoushka tradition teaches us
            to explore all the different personas
            on the wheel
The extent to which we recognize
            and realize in ourselves
                        all of these sexual personas
            is the extent to which
                        we have a full, balanced sexual life

This was but one of the teachings
            given by the shaman
            before closing with the Sacred Pipe Ceremony
                        to give thanks
                        to all the powers/energies/essences/beauty
                                    for being present and guiding us
                                    during the sexual teachings

6. Massage as Meditation

The body is a temple
                        for the spirit
            This has long been a mystical tenet

The physical body is more than a tool
                        to accomplish physical tasks

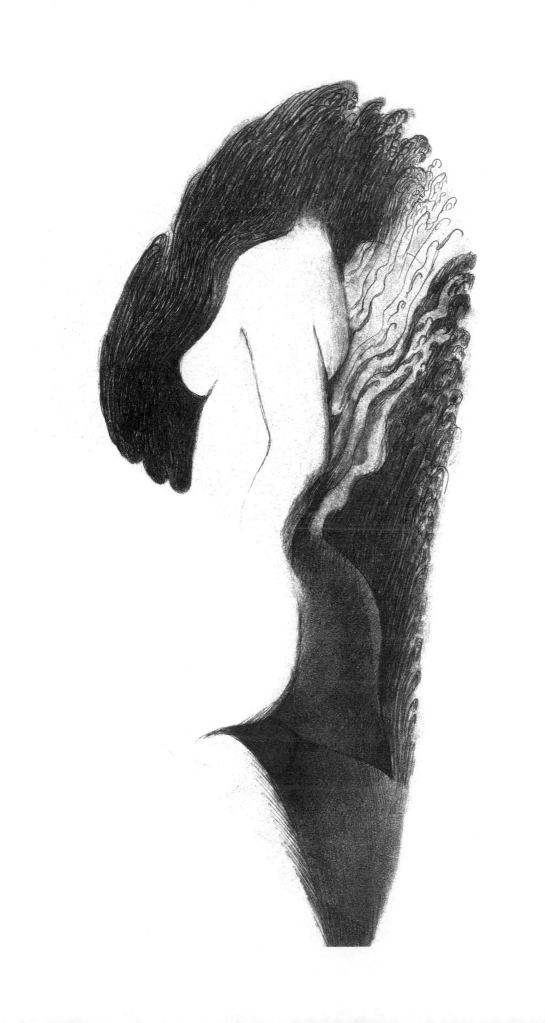

It is more than a resting place
for the mind
By being aware, by focusing
on our physical sensations
whatever
wherever they are
we are more able to bring ourselves
into the present
In this presence,
is where
we are more likely to find
our spiritual dimensions

It is incredibly simple:
we quiet the mind
by placing our awareness on the physical
and we touch the spiritual
which brings us back
to the meaning and the beauty
of physical existence

For me, human touch
was the meditation
that brought me back most
to my spiritual dimension

A formal name for human touch is
massage
Massage, actually, usually, at least for me,
is a two-person meditation
Learning to give and to receive massage
is a training in being present:
our hands touch the body
we allow our body to be touched
with awareness
with attentiveness
with mindfulness
It was here
in the study of massage
that I discovered/evolved
my own, personal,
contemporary form of meditation

Massage is a dance
between two
—one active, one receptive
Giving massage, truly giving
is like sculpting:
smoothing away the rough edges
to allow the beauty within

           to be revealed
Receiving massage, truly receiving
      is opening ourselves
         to experience
      the totality of ourself
This is the meditation of,
         the art of massage

Massage is ancient
      The forms are varied
      What makes them *massage*
         is the patterned touch
The patterns
      usually are done with the hands
      sometimes with the feet
      occasionally with the elbows or knees
      occasionally with other parts of the body
The patterns can be
      deep, firm
      light, delicate
      vigorous, intense
      gentle, subtle
      slow, still
      rapid, quick
The emphasis can be on the
      skin
      muscles
      fascia which surround the muscles
      internal organs
      joints
      blood circulation
      lymph circulation
      pressure points
      energy fields
         within and/or exterior to the physical body
The intent can be
      more physical, such as
         to reduce muscular tension
         to assist tissue healing
         to detoxify, to cleanse
      more psychological/emotional, such as
         to open up, to release
            blocked/repressed/suppressed feelings of
               sadness
               contentment
               fearfulness
               anger
               joy
               sexual arousal

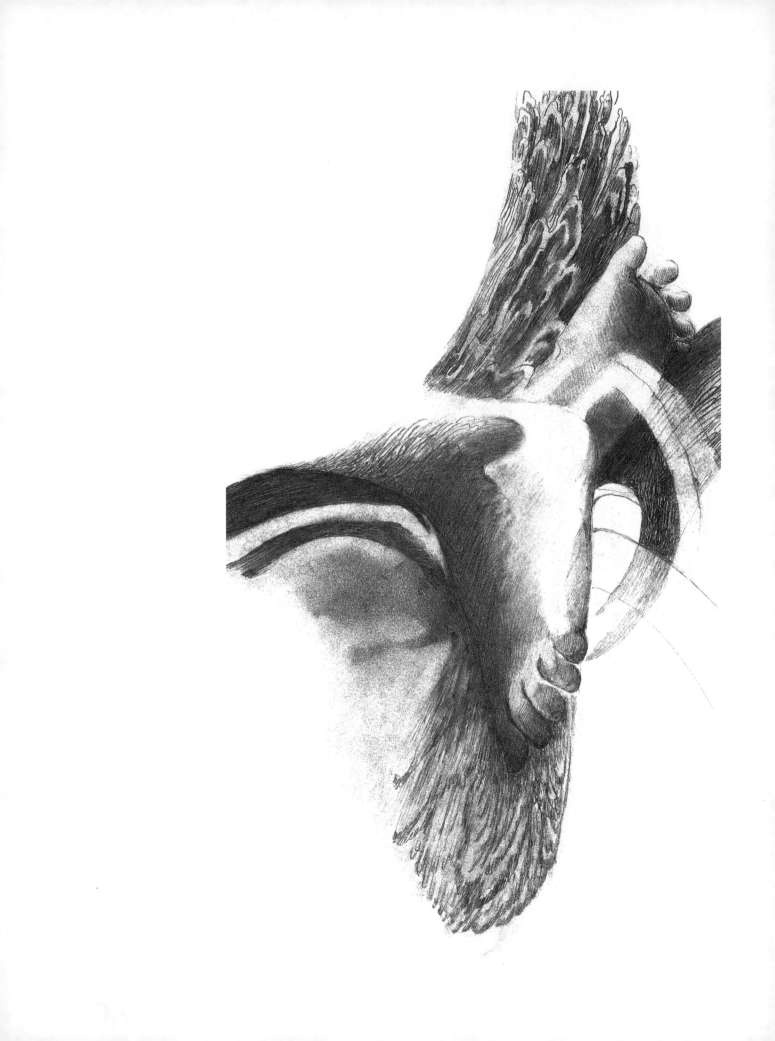

Many massage forms
        have other names than *massage*
    many are forms from other centuries, other cultures
    many are current
        developments/modifications/adaptations
    many are so synthesized
        they constitute
        a new, contemporary cultural form themselves
but all are basically
    one person touching another
    in patterned methods
        usually, potentially,
            with awareness
            with attentiveness
            with mindfulness

As a meditation,
    massage brings us into direct contact
        with each other's
            mind/body/spirit/emotion
Two people open themselves, potentially,
    to intimacy
    to a common union, to communion
    to a depth of emotional connection
        that can be experienced
            usually only
        when making love:
            vulnerability
            sensitivity
            respect
            appreciation
            merging together energetically
The only real difference
    between a massage and making love
    is that massage,
        as it is taught most of the time
            in professional trainings
            and in personal growth classes,
    does not involve
        genital touching and orgasm, intentionally

In my professional massage training
    I learned a donut massage
        —there was a hole in the middle
            physically and emotionally
    Massage techniques were taught
        for every part of the exterior physical body
        except for *down there*
            between the legs
            (Most massage schools
                exclude female breasts,

some exclude the buttocks,
some exclude even more)
All human feelings/emotions were accepted:
if there are tears, good, let them flow
release the sadness
if there is anger, good,
pound on pillows
express it through sounds in your voice
release the suppressed emotion
All human feelings/emotions were accepted
except for one, basic, primary one:
sexual

But sooner or later,
if we touch other human beings
personally and/or professionally
we will have choices to make
regarding sexual feelings
choices about
how to respond to others' sexual feelings/emotions
when and how to express our own
sexual feelings/emotions

Most of us, most of the time
make an unconscious choice: we suppress

However, to the extent that we
suppress/repress/deny/demean
our emotional dimensions
is the extent to which
we limit our spiritual dimensions

Moreover, the more we suppress/repress/deny/demean
our emotional dimensions,
the more likely that
suppressed emotions
will be expressed in abusive ways

Somewhere along the way
most of us came to a belief, a decision
that the only option to
sexual suppression/control
is
uncontrollable, animalistic desire/passion/lust
There *are* more options, more conscious choices
This is what the tantric, Taoist,
· and Quodoushka teachings
as well as massage
are about:
the transformation of energy

For me personally
    it was the meditation of massage
        more than any other form
    that brought me face-to-face
        with my sexuality
    Every time I gave or received
        a massage,
        the potential for sexual feelings
        was there
    The more powerful, the more impactful the massage,
        the more the potential
    regardless of the other's
        gender, age, physical appearance,
        or nature of our relationship
    This is where I learned most
        how to transform the energy of sexual feelings,
        and thus to be more in conscious choice

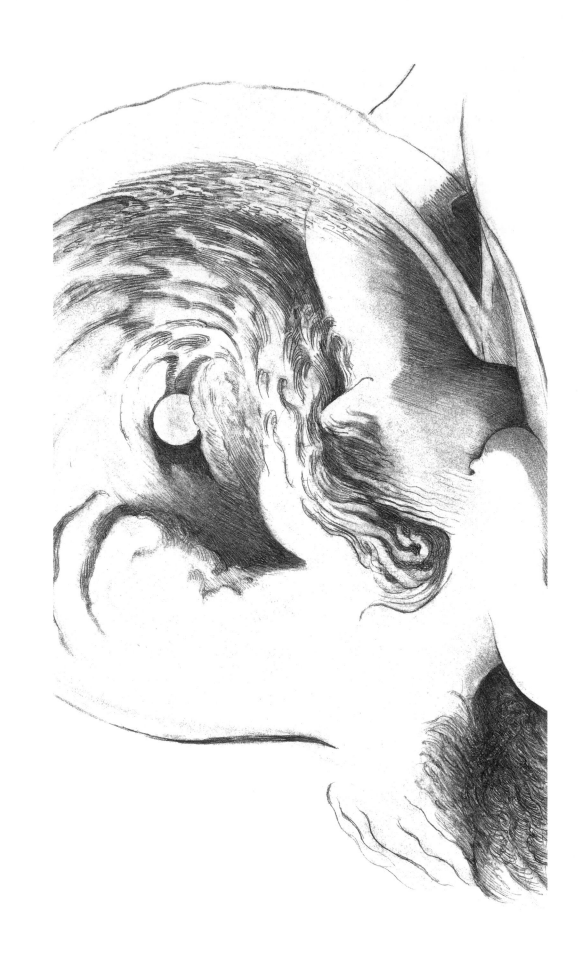

III Orgasm As Transformation

7. Signposts

What we don't need is another
    dogma
    or another rigid belief system
        to become attached to
        to defend
        to attack
        to be politically correct about
        to create a religious group around
Dogmas and other rigid belief systems
        limit us
    they have all the answers
    we no longer question them
    we no longer live our experience
        we live our beliefs, lifelessly
On the other hand, without conceptual frameworks,
        a multitude of events/experiences
        appear unrelated
    we don't see/feel/sense/hear
        the meaning of it all
Somewhere
        between dogma and meaning*less*ness
    there is
        meaning*ful*ness

The following is a set of signposts
        in which I find meaning

Even with the signposts, though,
there are, along the way,
unpaved roads
washed-out bridges
quicksand
Sometimes these signs
use the same term
that other maps use
but mean different things/directions
and very often use a different term
than other maps use
to mean the same things/directions
It all gets terribly confusing
at times

But at least signposts
for me
confirm that someone is seeking

Sacred Orgasms proposes
a paradigm shift
from the contemporary Western predominant
points of view
both scientific and religious
These are the central concepts:
1. We are more than a physical body
2. Orgasms are an energetic experience
and sexual orgasms
are only one type of orgasm
3. What we call our spiritual and our sexual aspects
are not only
not in opposition,
they are mutually enhancing

The conceptual framework/paradigm
that follows
embellishes these three ideas
The framework is
a way of holding it all together,
a way of understanding,
of bringing meaning to personal experiences
The framework
is *not* a synthesis
of others'
traditions, teachings, concepts, information
The concepts and meditations are designed for people
living in a modern culture
in modern times
The framework is an evolution
continuing to evolve

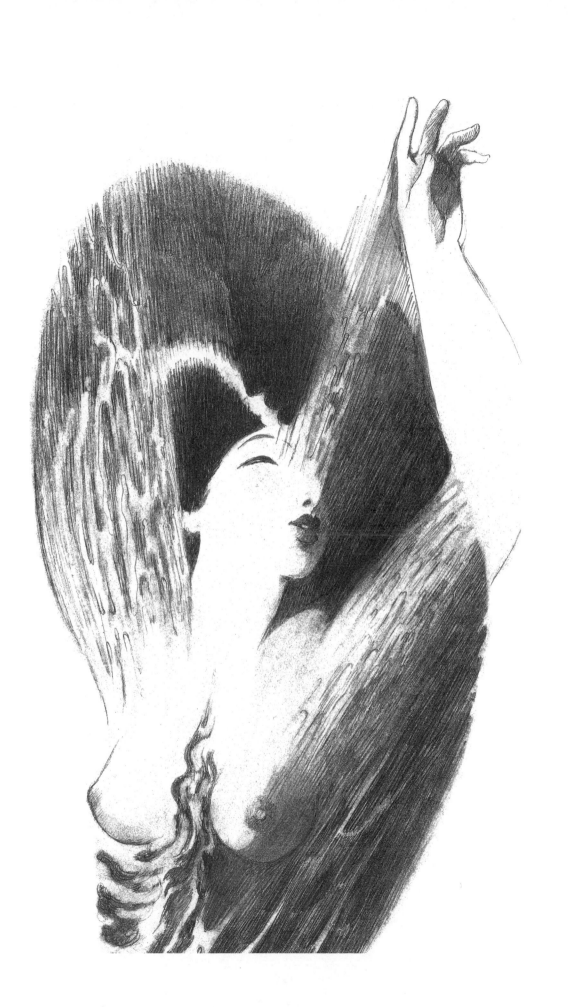

and is far more complex
than it appears here
There are many more functions than described
and the structures vary
depending on the circumstances
and phases of development
The framework may appear to be static
It definitely is not
The descriptions
are not always applicable to each of us
during our many different
possible phases of development
(This is one of the reasons
there are so many different
descriptions/interpretations
by different frameworks
of energy
and subtle energy systems)

What follows is
a theoretical model,
a conceptual framework,
a paradigm
for some of us some of the time
describing what a human being is / potentially can be
describing what orgasm is / potentially can be

8. The Anatomy of a Being

What we call a human being
is more than a physical body
In *Sacred Orgasms*
what we are
is a more-or-less integration
of several systems

Some of the systems
at least some of the time
appear as a shape similar to a physical body
Some have no semblance to a body shape
This is why the word *system*
rather than *body*
(Some frameworks describe layers of energy fields
In some cases, these fields are likely to be
emanations
of some of the following systems
but are not discussed here)

In outline form, this is a human being:

A. the soul system
  - soul
  - soul centers
  - sphere
  - core

B. the seven incarnated systems
  a. the six subtle energy systems
    - spirit body
    the five "engine" systems
      - light body
      - chakra system
      - resonance system
      - kundalini system
      - resource system
  b. • physical body

All of these systems
      can, in a sense, co-occupy
         the same space at the same time
           with each other
         as only the physical body is physical matter
We might also say the systems
      coexist or *interpenetrate*

To simplify descriptions,
      the physical body parts/areas
         are the labels to locate the other systems
The physical body area, however,
      may or may not have a functional relationship
        with the other identified system

The Soul System

Prior to incarnating
      the soul is a single unit
After the soul merges with the sperm-egg union
      in the uterus,
      the soul differentiates into four primary parts
  - the soul, in the navel area
  - the ten soul centers, from the pelvic floor
    to a couple of feet above the head
  - the sphere, surrounding all the systems
    of a human being
  - the core, connecting from
    the bottom of the sphere
    to the top of the sphere,
    which are the two ends of the being

THE ANATOMY OF A BEING

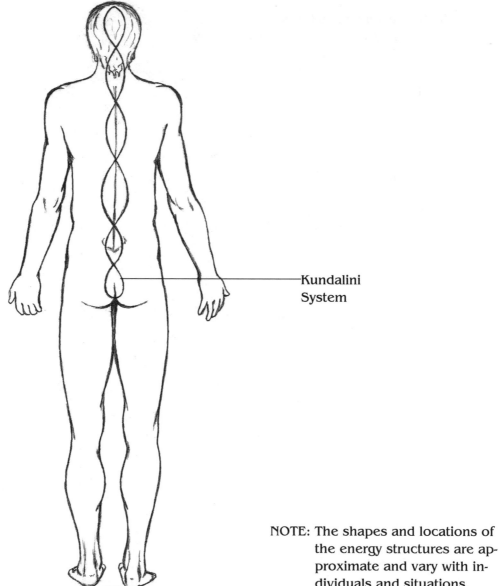

Kundalini
System

NOTE: The shapes and locations of
the energy structures are ap-
proximate and vary with individuals and situations.

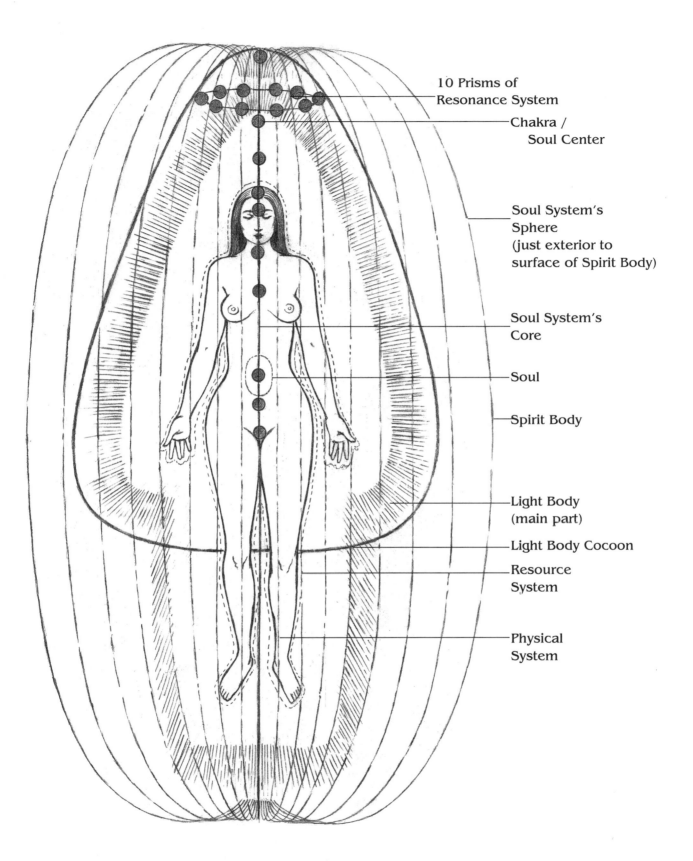

10 Prisms of
Resonance System

Chakra /
Soul Center

Soul System's
Sphere
(just exterior to
surface of Spirit Body)

Soul System's
Core

Soul

Spirit Body

Light Body
(main part)

Light Body Cocoon

Resource
System

Physical
System

The Soul

This is the operations center
                    of the soul system
        This is the center
                    of our be-ness,
                the heart of our wholeness,
                the part of us that is
                            God/Source/Goddess
The soul is oval shaped,
                extending about three inches
                            above and below the navel
The soul's initial primary function
            is to merge
                    with the fertilized egg
        and provide the seeds of what we call *life*
            for the physical body
As each of our soul centers (below)
            become fully developed through our lifetime,
            the soul becomes more and more capable
                    of its full potential
                            in this incarnation

The Soul Centers

A human being has
                ten soul centers
            distributed along the midline of the body
                    from the pelvic floor
                    to about an arm's length above the head
They are at the same spaces as
                the focal points of the chakras
            but structurally, functionally, and energetically
                    distinct from the chakras

The soul centers serve, in a sense,
                as the soul's regional managers
                        of the different sections
                        of the seven incarnated systems
            Other possible names for the soul centers
                    might be
                the knowledge centers
                the wisdom centers
            names which imply some of the centers' functions

Developing sequentially up the midline,
            the first soul center,
                    at the center of the pelvic floor,
                    starts automatically at birth

The second soul center,
> midway between the pelvic floor
>> and the navel,
> begins automatically to develop
>> at puberty

The third soul center,
> at the navel area,
> begins automatically to develop
>> near the end of puberty

From then on,
> full development of each soul center
>> is basically dependent on
> which soul centers were fully developed
>> in previous incarnations

and on
> personal endeavor in this incarnation

And this full development
> is the primary focus of
>> the eight integration meditations,
> which use orgasm
>> as the most effective
>>> energy generator
>> for such an endeavor

Then, when all ten soul centers
> are fully developed,
the soul can function as God/Source/Goddess
> to the extent possible
>> in incarnated form

Said another way:
> God/Source/Goddess cannot incarnate
> So when we fully develop
>> our ten soul centers,
> we can function as God could
>>> on the physical plane
>> if God could incarnate

In *Sacred Orgasms*, the soul centers are
> the key
> the journey
to our wholeness,
to our greatest incarnated potential
And orgasm is our vehicle

The Sphere

The soul system's sphere
> is a continuous current of energy
> enveloping all other parts of the soul system
> and the seven incarnated systems,

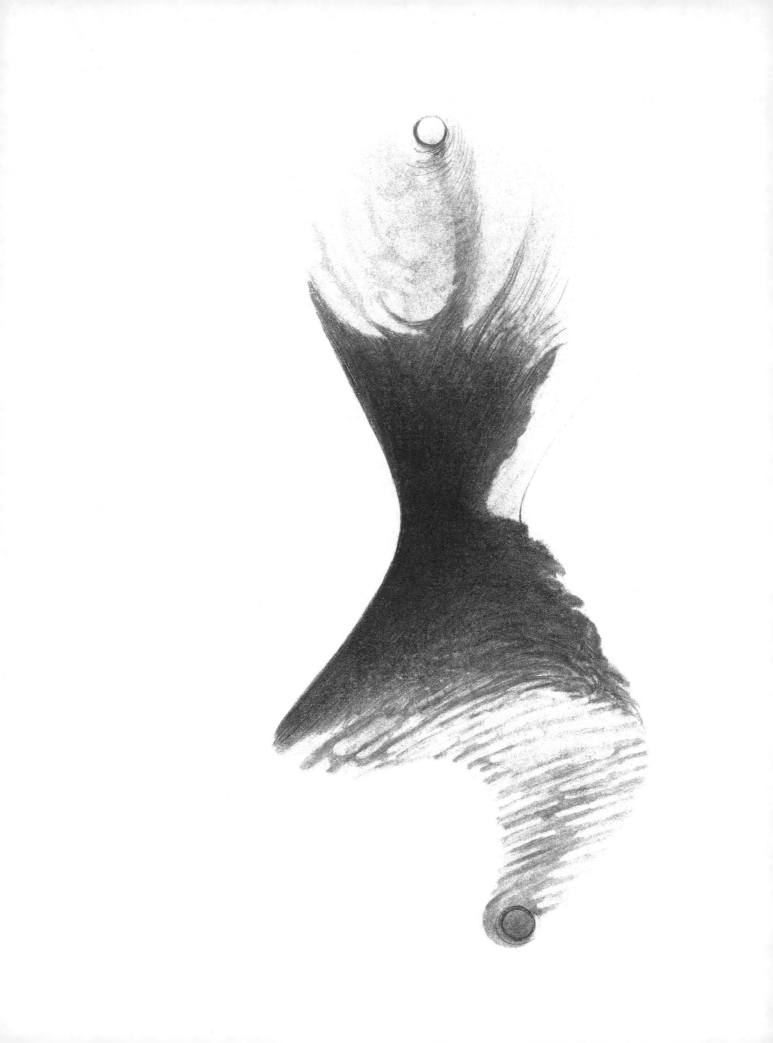

This large, oval-shaped sphere
    and everything interior to it
constitute the being,
    in our case,
    the human being
Our sphere
    is the parameter
    delineating us from any other being

The Core

The soul system's core is a current of energy
    connecting the two ends of the sphere,
    thus connecting the two ends of the being
The soul at the navel area
    and the ten soul centers
    and the central operating systems
      of the seven incarnated systems
    lie along the path of this current
      and are thus connected

The Incarnated Systems

Being incarnated is
    a physical body
    with six other systems
      —the spirit body being the most subtle,
    the physical body being the most dense

Using driving a car as an analogy,
    we might think of the seven incarnated systems like this:

    the spirit body is like
      the driver of a car,
        making the choices in direction
        and speed

    the five "engine" systems are like
      the engine-distributor-carburetor of a car,
        implementing the spirit body's
        choices

    and the physical body is like
      the transmission and the wheels,
      where the rubber
        hits the road

The Spirit Body

The spirit body
      is an oval-shaped system that encompasses
          all the other incarnated systems
     and extends approximately
         two feet below the feet to
         two feet above the head
     (The soul system's sphere
         is just exterior to the exterior surface
           of the spirit body)

There are two main functions
     of the spirit body
When there is an orgasm,
       any kind of orgasm,
      primordial incarnated energy is
         generated/created/originated/developed
     This type of energy can easily be transformed
       by any incarnated system
       for use by that system
The spirit body is where
      any not-yet-used primordial incarnated energy
       is temporarily suspended

The second main function of the spirit body
     concerns the informational and emotional aspects
      of an experience
Sometimes, after the resource system (discussed later)
     separates the purely informational aspect
      to be stored as memory,
     the emotional part reattaches
      to the codified information,
      as in the grasping and avoiding
        of attachments,
      as in emotional
        blockage/repression/suppression
During orgasm
     the spirit body can unstick
        in conjunction with the light body
      at least some of the attachments
This is the how
     in the why
       most of us most of the time
     are so emotionally content
      after an orgasm
The sometimes tears and crying
      after an orgasm
     are rarely due to sadness and grief
     during lovemaking or masturbation

The bursting out in laughter
            here is not from a joke
These are emotional releases
            which the spirit body facilitates

            The Light Body

The light body is the managing system
            of the five "engine" systems
which are the incarnated systems that
            in a sense, provide the fuel
            for the spirit body to accomplish
                in the physical body
            what the spirit body has chosen

When seen
        this system looks like
                a body of light
        and is thus named
The light is bright and with colors,
        the color of which depending on
                at least to some extent
        the mental-emotional tone of the person

The light body's primary structure has a shape
        similar to the physical body,
                extending about one foot
                exterior to the physical body,
        and permeates the physical body throughout
Inside the physical body,
        the light body flows through
                a vast network of minute channels
Some call these channels the *nadis*
                (pronounced *nah' dees*)
        of which there are about 72,000
                    according to yogic texts
Some of these channels are
                the acupuncture meridians

The light body's principal function
        is to carry/distribute energy
                throughout the physical body
The light body serves two additional,
            sometimes critical, functions:
        what we might call extraordinary endurance
                and extraordinary strength
We wonder how in heroic rescues
                or other emergencies
        the body can work far longer

and/or far more powerfully
than in usual, everyday life
It is the light body
that has been
tapped into / utilized / drawn upon

One part of the light body
is especially important
for the eight integration meditations
that follow:
The cocoon
extends from approximately
two feet below the pelvis to
two feet above the head
and approximately two feet exterior to all parts
of the torso and head
This part of the light body is
a continuous current of energy
that functions as a filtering parameter
allowing only certain energies inside
to the chakras and kundalini system
and other parts
of the subtle energy systems

The Chakra System

Chakras, probably,
are the most described / discussed / pursued
of the subtle energy systems
in esoteric/mystical/metaphysical/spiritual
traditions

Each chakra is
a single spinning vortex, initially
In later stages of development
some of the chakras
are two or three spinning vortexes
The spinning vortex has an appearance
sort of like a cone
Personally, I am more likely to feel
the smaller ends
which are the area of energetic focalization
and are more or less along the core of
the physical body

In *Sacred Orgasms*
there are ten principal chakras
located from
just above the pelvic floor

to about two feet above
the top of the head
(In the diagram, the location
of the focal points of the chakras
and the soul centers
is indicated by the same disk
since they are basically
in the same location)

Many esoteric teachings
focus on seven or five principal chakras,
all of which are usually considered between
the pelvic floor and
the top of the head
Without meditations on the three chakras
(and three soul centers)
above the top of the head, however,
the soul system is far less likely
to become fully developed

Chakras, in a sense,
are the digestion system
for the other subtle energy systems
The main function of the chakras
most of the time for most of us
is to
transform/convert/transubstantiate/transmute
forms of energy
into other usable forms of energy
for the subtle energy systems

The Resonance System

The resonance system is a set of
ten spinning vortexes,
which I call prisms
These appear similar to chakras
but unlike the basically stationary chakras,
the prisms
move throughout the other six systems
within the light body cocoon
facilitating the cocoon
in its filtering function

The resonance system's principal function,
similar to the chakras',
is transformation of energies
into energy forms the other subtle energy systems
can utilize

The Kundalini System

Kundalini (pronounced *coon dah lee´ nee*)
    like *chakra*
    is another word from Sanskrit
Kundalini, the term,
    is used many different ways
   and sometimes in the West
     the kundalini system is confused
      with the chakra system
   Both systems
    are along the midline of the body, and
   both systems' main function
    is to transform energy
     into forms of energy
    usable by other subtle energy systems

Their structures, however,
    are very different
The kundalini system,
    as I am using the term here,
   is a continuous current of energy
   ascending and descending
    in two wavelike patterns,
    basically along the spinal column

The Resource System

The resource system for most of us
   is what we call memory
    (that can be accessed
    by the physical body brain)

Appearing as
    a soft, white-light glow
this system surrounds
   the entire physical body surface,
   usually from just beneath the skin
    to the exterior of the physical body
     about half an inch

The resource system's main function usually
   is to serve as
   a storehouse of information
The resource system
   codifies the informational aspects of all our
    thoughts, inner images,
    sensations, feelings/emotions,
    and any other experiences,

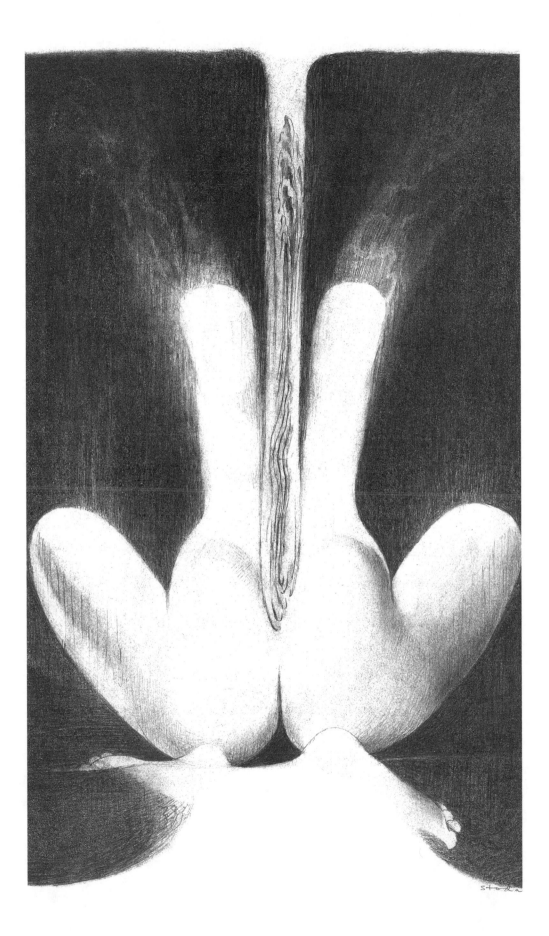

usually separating the emotional aspect
to flow freely,
unattached to the informational aspect
Then as needed,
this system can access and retrieve
the information
if, and this is a major *if,*
emotional blockage/repression/suppression
does not interfere
(As indicated before, in orgasm
the spirit body facilitates separating
the informational aspect stuck to
the emotional aspect)

The Physical Body

The physical body system is a structure of
muscles, bones, nerves, arteries, veins,
organs, glands,
and so on
This is the incarnated system
that most of us think of as "me"
The physical body is obviously
where the rubber hits the road
Obviously, we would have little effect
in the physical world
without a physical body

For the other six incarnated systems,
obvious no longer applies
Unfortunately, without obvious, observable, discernible
objects or events
we can slip easily into woo-woo land
Woo-woo is *not* another spiritual, Eastern term
like wu-wei
Woo-woo
is nomenclature for
spaced-out
ungrounded
unfounded
nonreality
I have wondered/worried
if all this is a woo-woo framework
My orgasms,
my own wide variety of orgasmic experiences,
however, are what kept bringing me back to
"maybe the paradigm is valid"
—the orgasm sensations are real!

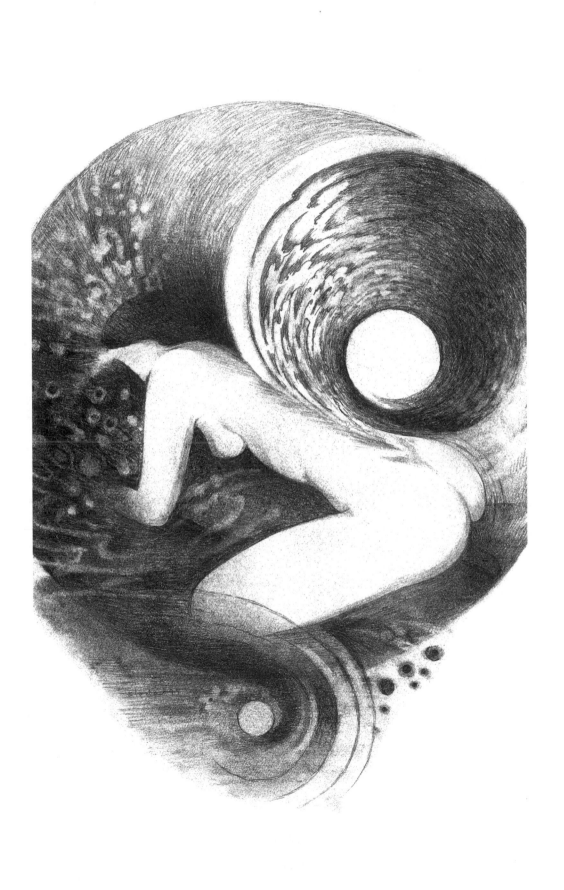

9. The Four Types of Orgasms

As we shift

               if we choose to shift
          to a point of view that
          we are not only a physical body,
      our definition/model of orgasm
              might shift as well

Sexual orgasm can be

          a special, wonderful experience
      Sexual orgasm can also be
          a teacher
          a prototype
          an indication
              of what orgasm *in general* is like
     A pelvic-floor-contractions definition of orgasm,
              however, does not explain
          some of the out-of-the-ordinary orgasms
                  presented earlier
Here is a broader definition
          (the social sciences
               would call it a *conceptual definition*
               rather than an *operational definition*):
Orgasm
     is an event where
     two or more vibratory patterns change
          so that they resonate with each other,
     and a new vibratory pattern occurs
          which consists of
               the initial vibratory patterns
               plus the vibratory pattern of
                    primordial incarnated energy

Primordial incarnated energy (my complex term)

          is one of ten types of energy
               used by the incarnated systems
       This type is
          undifferentiated, not-yet-formed energy
               that is the energy best suited
               to develop all ten soul centers
      All types of orgasm
          are a major, easily available source
               of this primordial incarnated energy
          which is needed in immense quantities
          in our soul center development endeavors

Energy generation

          is the emphasis in this definition

in contrast
to the predominant contemporary focus
on *tension release*
Both characterizations are valid
The *Sacred Orgasms* definition, however,
supplies the key to the answer
of the question of
why orgasms are sacred:
All orgasms generate primordial incarnated energy
Primordial incarnated energy is the most beneficial
means for full development
of all the soul centers
When all our soul centers are
fully developed and integrated,
our everyday consciousness has direct access
to our individual soul,
which is a part of God/Source/Goddess
—the central operating system soul
for all existence
Thus,
orgasm is the most direct route
for our everyday consciousness
to be in direct, conscious connection
with God

This is an oversimplification
But it says that we are always at-one with God
though we are not all
consciously aware of our at-one-ment
This paradigm also implies
that any tradition that denies or prohibits
sexuality and orgasm
in effect robs us
of our most direct route to God
Our sexuality and our orgasm are a vehicle
back to the Garden

. . .

In *Sacred Orgasms*
sexual orgasm is but one
of four types of orgasm
though sexual orgasm is the key
to the other types
Until we experience a sexual orgasm,
our incarnated systems literally do not know
what an orgasm is
Sexual orgasm, thus, is
the initiating teacher

Conceptually, there are four types of orgasm
    because four of the systems
        in the preceding anatomy of a human being
    are capable of orgasm as just defined
These four systems are
    • the physical body
    • the light body
    • the spirit body
    • the soul system
There are, however,
    far more than four types of orgasmic experiences
        as indicated in the earlier descriptions
        of different out-of-the-ordinary orgasms
    and many of these orgasms may not feel sexual
        or occur in a sexual context
            (depending on how we think of *sex*)
An individual orgasm can
    be of only one of the types of orgasm
        or a combination of two or more types,
    occur in all of a system
        or concentrated in areas of a system,
    and vary in intensity
        from an earlier orgasm of the same type
So, four different types of orgasm
    does not mean
    four different distinct orgasmic experiences

In the following descriptions,
    to comprehend the orgasm typology
    we would best temporarily suspend
        our distinctions between
            sexual, spiritual, and mystical

Sexual Orgasm

A sexual orgasm
    is what most of us mean
        when we say *orgasm*
    Thus sexual orgasm is the name I use for
        a physical body orgasm
As already described,
    this is the pelvic-floor-contractions orgasm
    often resulting from physical stimulation of the
        clitoris, G spot, penis, and/or prostate areas
            possibly other areas for some of us
    Ejaculation is common with male bodies
        but not so common with female bodies

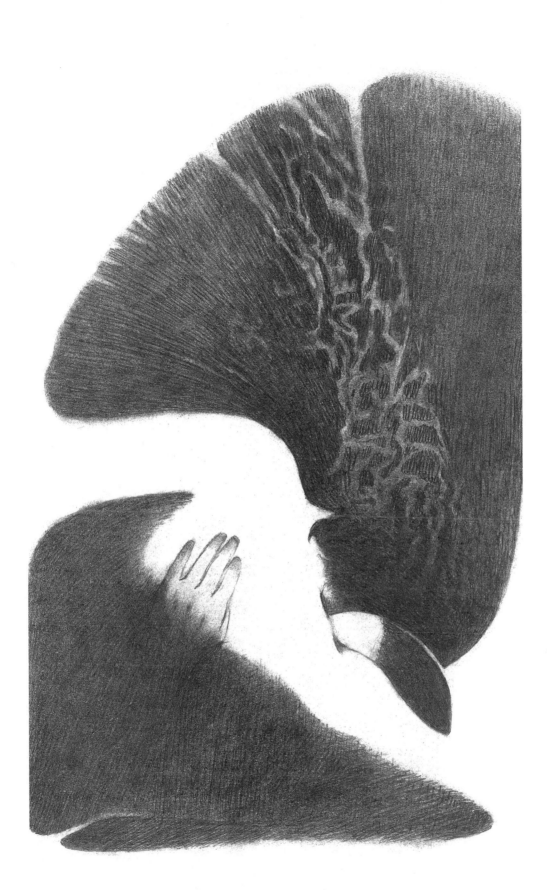

though now that science has discovered
the fact that female bodies can ejaculate,
many more women are likely
to learn to ejaculate
(Note: science treats
ejaculation and sexual orgasm as
two distinct physiological phenomena
which can occur in conjunction)

The other three types of orgasm
may have effects on the physical body
but the orgasm is not occurring
in the physical body itself
Minor or extensive physical body movements
can occur
Subtle or intense sensations can be felt
sometimes labeled as
pleasurable, electric, explosive, lit up
But unless an orgasm is
a combination of types including a sexual orgasm,
pelvic floor contractions and an ejaculation
are not likely to be
in the orgasmic experience
of the other three types

Light Body Orgasm

A light body orgasm
occurs only in the light body
However, since the light body functions closely
with the other four "engine" systems
(chakras, resonance system,
kundalini system, and
resource system)
a light body orgasm might be focused
in the areas where these other systems are,
such as a little explosion
in the heart chakra area in the chest
A light body orgasm can also occur
throughout the whole light body

What some call a *total body orgasm*
is probably a light body orgasm
and sexual orgasm combined
This is the not-always-mythical orgasm
where rockets are bursting in air
where the whole body
is consumed in rapture

Romanticized storytelling
　　　　might employ such imagery,
　　　but human beings are indeed capable
　　　of such intense energetic experiences

Spirit Body Orgasm

A spirit body orgasm
　　　is focused in the whole spirit body
　　　or in the head area

What some call a *valley orgasm*
　　　　is probably one kind
　　　　　of spirit body orgasm
　　　Here an individual or partners
　　　　literally relax deeply
　　　　　into waves of pleasure

Making broad generalizations,
　　　many light body orgasms might be characterized
　　　　as *energetic*
　　　while comparatively,
　　　　tranquil might apply
　　　　　to many spirit body orgasms

Soul Orgasm

A soul orgasm
　　　is experienced in every part of the being
　　　　　or
　　　just in the soul (in the navel area)

Throughout the ages
　　　many major mystical experiences
　　　　　may have been soul orgasms
In this type of orgasm
　　　our energetic patterns are the same
　　　as God's energetic patterns
　　　　　just at far less intensity
This is why these orgasms are called
　　　mystical experiences

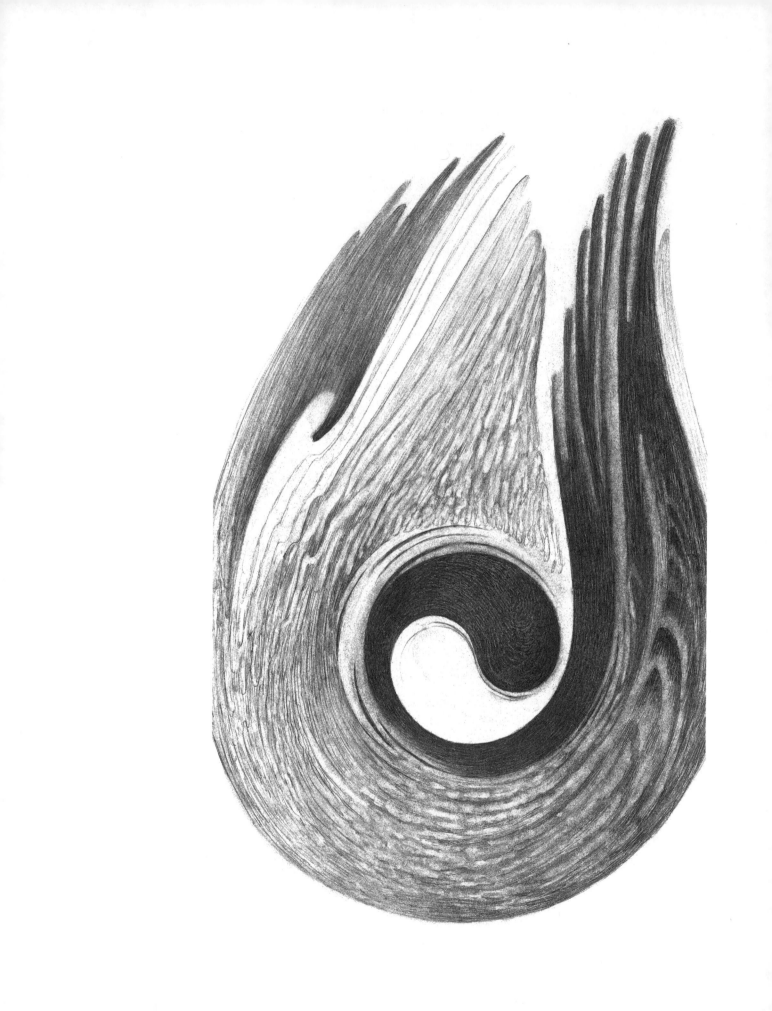

10. The Two Functions of Orgasm

In this framework
      each orgasm has two functions

One function of an orgasm
        that most of us would think of is
pleasure
        Not only physical pleasure, though
Orgasms can also be
          emotionally satisfying
          mentally stimulating
          and spiritually fulfilling
        All this is dependent
             at least to some extent
          on consensuality
          on no mitigating health conditions
          and no mitigating emotional conditions
             such as dishonest communications

      Note also that
      the pleasurable sensations of other types of orgasm
        may feel nothing at all like
          sexual orgasm pleasure

A second function of orgasm is
           transformation
        a term used throughout *Sacred Orgasms*
        and in various ways

Basically in this paradigm
      transformation means
          the converting of one form of energy
          into another form of energy
        The physical body digests/converts/transforms
          food into energy
        The chakras digest/convert/transform
          energy into forms of energy
          that other subtle energy systems can use
        And so on

More central to *Sacred Orgasms*
        is a particular type of transformation:
Under the section on tantra,
      we examined attachment
        —our emotional
          grasping and avoiding nature
Under the Taoist tradition
      we explored nonattachment
        conceived of as yielding and wu wei

In the Quodoushka tradition
being able to live life from any position
on the wheel
is nonattachment
Under the section on massage as meditation,
hands touching our body
encouraging/facilitating/allowing
blocked/repressed/suppressed
feelings/emotions
to release
—this is going from attachment
to nonattachment

As presented earlier, the resource system
transforms an experience into two parts:
the informational aspect
(stored memory until needed)
and the emotional aspect
However, after their transformation
the two energies sometimes
become reattached
Then, as more and more informational
and emotional energies
remain stuck together,
density develops—we have attachment
Psychologically, we speak of
pushing someone's button
(pushing someone's density)
In the musculature
we speak of body armoring
Potentially, there is a major impact on our health
as the attached energies become
more and more dense
Density
limits / slows down / constricts / restricts
the flow of energy
in both the physical body
and its energetic double, the light body
Density, eventually, results in
dis-ease and illness
in varying degrees in various ways
During orgasm,
the spirit body can transform the stuckness
in a way that separates the emotional energy
from the informational energy
Orgasm, in a sense,
dissolves the density
This can happen during sexual orgasms
and more so with
the other three types of orgasms

Thus, basically, generally,
      orgasms mean greater health
            greater well-being
            greater vibrancy

With all four types of orgasm
            on an ongoing basis,
     our ten soul centers and soul system can become
           fully developed
and our soul can integrate
        our soul system with our incarnated systems
When we have this full development
         of our being,
      we have thus transformed our whole being
         into having the ability
     to transform stuck energies
         with intent
Here we are able to transform
         (as discussed in the Introduction
             to *The Essential Tantra*)
     the poison of the poisonous plant
         into knowledge,
         into energy to nurture and heal all

Such a full development
         of our being,
   is the basic long-term purpose
     of the following
         eight integration meditations

11. The Integration Meditations

The eight integration meditations
         are the cornerstone of *Sacred Orgasms*
     Here is where we embody
         the teachings

Integration
         means the integration of the soul system
            with the seven incarnated systems
    Always there is interaction
         between these two sets of systems
     but until the ten soul centers
         and the whole soul system
         are fully developed,
    the soul
         can manifest only in limited ways
            on the physical plane

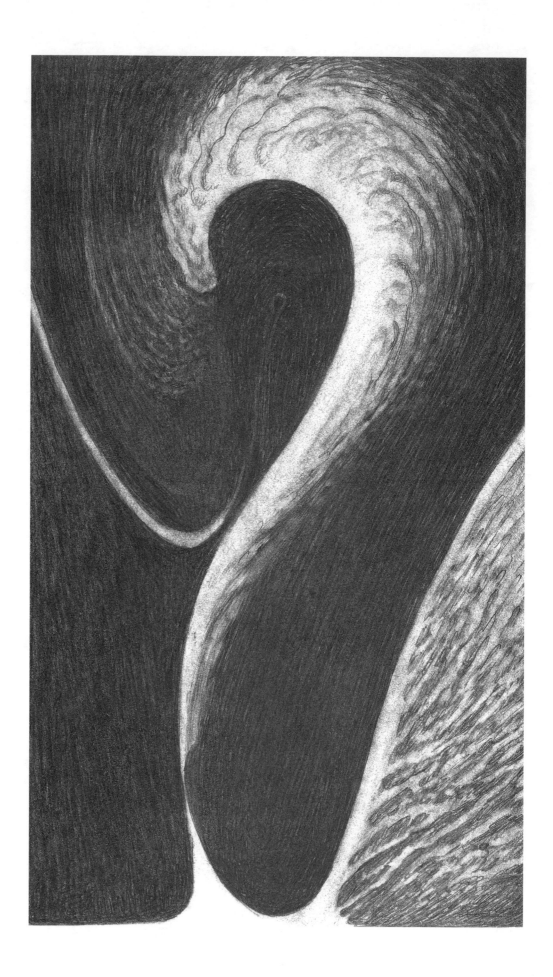

These meditations indeed place orgasm
                    at the center of the sacred circle
        Except for the sexual orgasm meditation
                    each meditation is a very mild form
                                of each type of orgasm,
                    so mild that some might say
                                nothing happened
        (Though when the eight meditations are practiced
                                over a long period of time,
                our capacity
                        to have more intense orgasms
                                increases for all four types)

The eight integration meditations are
                    two sets of four meditations:
                                the intensification meditations
                                and the orgasm meditations
They can be done
                in solitude,
                with another doing the same meditations, or
                with a group of others doing the same meditations
And the meditations are simple to do
                Except for the sexual orgasm meditation
                        each meditation may take only
                                    about one to two minutes
                        and requires only
                                    conscious awareness (attention),
                                    intent, and
                                    a familiarity with the preceding
                                            anatomy of the human being
        These meditations are definitely not visualizations
                When the directions refer to a place in a system
                        we are to actually feel/sense
                                the energy in that area,
                        not just imagine the anatomy illustration

A. The Intensification Meditations

This is a set of four intensification meditations
                    to tonify and expand the capacity
                    of all the systems

The first step is the same
                    for all four meditations:
                Place your conscious awareness
                        at the two ends of your being
                                (above your head and below your feet
                                where the anatomy diagram
                                        shows the top and the bottom

of the spirit body)
Sort of feel/sense upward about two or three feet
above the head
and downward about two or three feet
below the feet,
one end at a time
or both at the same time
Once you feel/sense the two ends,
shift your conscious awareness
to the next step

Indications for the completion of the second step
vary from person to person
and time to time
We might
feel a subtle movement of energy,
have a spontaneous larger inhalation,
have an obvious, sudden movement
of our torso muscles,
have an intuition that the meditation
is complete
There's no set cue
If nothing seems to happen
after a couple of minutes
start with step 1 again
If nothing seems to happen
after a few attempts
go to the next meditation
Generally, once we become familiar with the meditations,
a half a minute to about two minutes
might be a usual duration
for each of the four meditations
Compared to many other styles of meditation,
these are short
Simply complete each meditation
and move on to the next

Physical Body Intensification Meditation

1. Place your conscious awareness
in the two ends of your being
(above your head and below your feet)

2. Place your conscious awareness
in two points of the physical body:
the center top of your head and
the center of your pelvic floor
Continue until you sense a completion

"Engine" Systems Intensification Meditation

1. Place your conscious awareness
    in the two ends of your being
        (above your head and below your feet)

2. Place your conscious awareness
    in everything within your light body cocoon,
        extending from about two feet below
            the pelvic floor
        to about two feet above the head
        and about two feet exterior
            to all parts of the torso.
    Continue until you sense a completion

Spirit Body Intensification Meditation

1. Place your conscious awareness
    in the two ends of your being
        (above your head and below your feet)

2. Place your conscious awareness
    in the whole length of the soul system's core,
        the energy current
        going through the center of the being,
            connecting the two ends
            of the being and the spirit body
    Continue until you sense a completion

Soul System Intensification Meditation

1. Place your conscious awareness
    in the two ends of your being
        (above your head and below your feet)

2. Place your conscious awareness
    in every part of your whole being
        while focusing your awareness
            in your soul system
    Continue until you sense a completion

B. The Orgasm Meditations

The paradigm in *Sacred Orgasms*
    has four systems capable of orgasm
    and thus four different types of orgasm
In this set of four meditations
    each type of orgasm is experienced

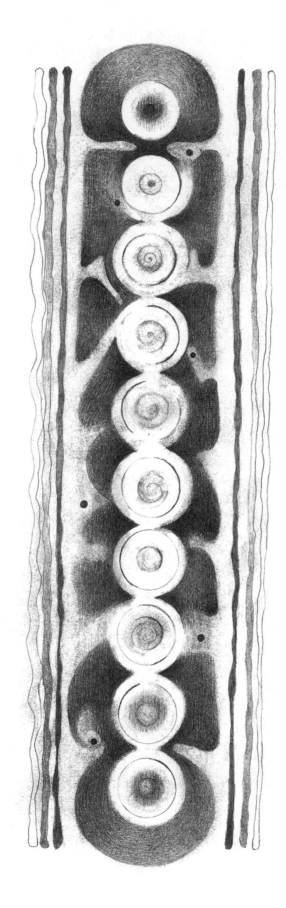

The primary purpose
>> of doing all four of these orgasms meditations
>>> as a sequence
>> is to generate an immense amount of
>>> primordial incarnated energy,
>>>> which is necessary to fully develop
>>>>> the soul centers and soul system

The physical body orgasm
>>> which I call a sexual orgasm
>> is done in any pattern
>>> with which you are already familiar,
>> masturbating by yourself
>> and/or making love with another
>>>> who is also doing the meditation
>>>>> at the same time

The other three types of orgasm
>>> are accomplished with intent
Intent here is a sort of
>>>> nonphysical doing
>>> While intent can involve
>>>>> mental images and thoughts,
>>>> the everyday mind is not what is doing
>>>>> the intending
>>>> The soul is the intending source
When you do the intending
>>> explore doing the intending
>>>> from the navel area
>>>>> not the physical navel
>>>>> but the soul
>>>>>> in the navel area, inside
>> If this method of intending
>>>> feels awkward,
>>> explore a more mental approach
>>> but know that intending
>>>> is far more than a mental exercise

These other three types of orgasm
>>> will likely be rather mild experiences,
>>>> nothing much like a sexual orgasm
>>>> and nothing much
>>>>> like a usual orgasm experience
>>>>> of these three others types
>>>>>> of orgasm
Moreover, these three orgasms
>>> are likely to feel similar in intensity
>>>> to the second step completion
>>>> of the previous intensification meditations
Remember, these are long-term practices

focusing on the transformation function
of orgasm
Orgasms are energy generators
Here we are employing
the full range of orgasms
to transform ourselves
into being all we can be
Practical by-products, however,
of doing these meditations on a long-term basis
could include
more intense sexual orgasms and
new and different pleasures
when making love and
when connecting energetically
with others

Sexual Orgasm Meditation

Stimulate the physical body
in any way
until you have a sexual orgasm

Light Body Orgasm Meditation

1. Place your conscious awareness
in every part of your five "engine" systems:
light body, chakra system,
resonance system, kundalini system,
and resource system
Continuing with step 1,
include step 2

2. Intend for your light body to have an orgasm

Spirit Body Orgasm Meditation

1. Place your conscious awareness
in every part of your spirit body
and the soul system's core
(the energy current connecting
the two ends of the spirit body)
Continuing with step 1,
include step 2

2. Intend for your spirit body to have an orgasm

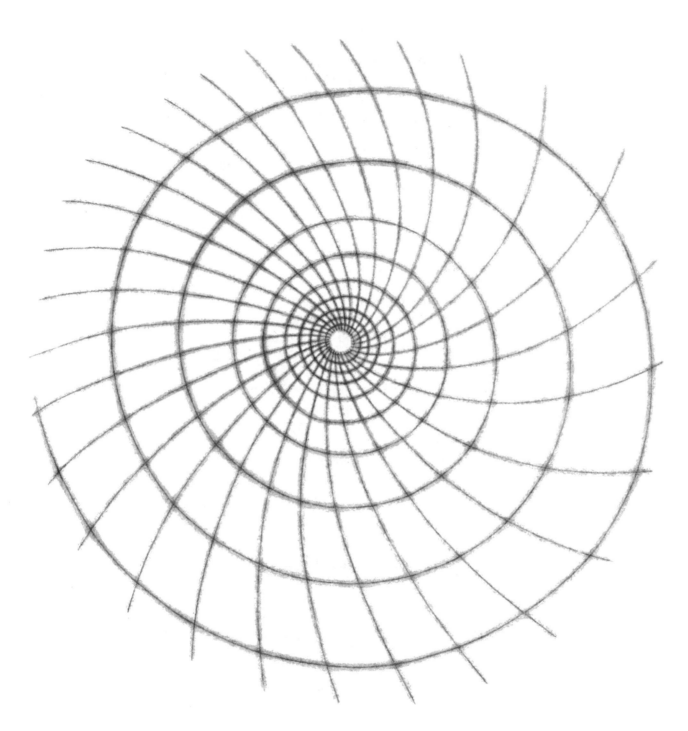

Diagram 3

Soul Center in Orgasm
(when all ten are developed)

Soul Orgasm Meditation

1. Place your conscious awareness
in every part of your being
Continuing with step 1,
include step 2

2. Place conscious awareness in soul system and
intend for your soul to have an orgasm

When to do the meditations:

Following an established pattern
for seven days a week
would be best
though by no means critical
Ideally, do one set of four in the morning
just after waking
and the other set of four in the evening
just prior to sleep
If such a pattern is not feasible,
try to have at least three hours
between the two sets
Whichever sets you do
for the earlier and later sessions
is your choice
Though it's advisable
to keep the pattern consistent
Also, explore possible sequences
within each set of four
until you find a pattern
that feels best for you

The integration meditations with another or others:

With the integration meditations
when meditating with another or others,
the most important guideline
is to have the intent of connection
with another or others
Be open to actually feeling
your energy fields combining
Be in physical proximity
While definitely an option,
physical touching
is not actually necessary

If you are doing the meditations
            with a sexual partner,
    you can include the orgasm meditations
            as a part of your lovemaking
    although communicate in some way
            so that both are focusing
    on the same type of orgasm at the same time
The sexual orgasm meditation can be
            during coitus,
            or with mutual noncoital stimulation,
            or with self-stimulation while having
                an intent of connection
                        with another or others
Simultaneous orgasms
            are by no means necessary
    Just wait until both have completed
                the same orgasm meditation
            before going to the next meditation
And if one of the orgasms does not occur for someone
            just continue with the series
It's best, however, not to skip over any of the meditations
            without attempting the meditation
    Thus should one or both partners
                not be in a lovemaking mood
    the meditations can always be done
                in solitude
Moreover, doing the meditations near someone else
            who is not doing the meditations
                    at the same time
            can interfere with the benefits
                of doing the meditations
    Again, find solitude space
                    for yourself

What to do with the energy from the meditation:

Our soul is far wiser
            than our everyday mind
    In these meditations
                simply let the soul do its thing
    Do not attempt
                to direct the resulting energy
    Forego any intent other than
                the intent in the orgasm meditation
    Forgo affirmations with the meditations
    If you wish,
            affirmations and other intents
                can be applied in orgasms
                which are not a part
                of these integration meditations

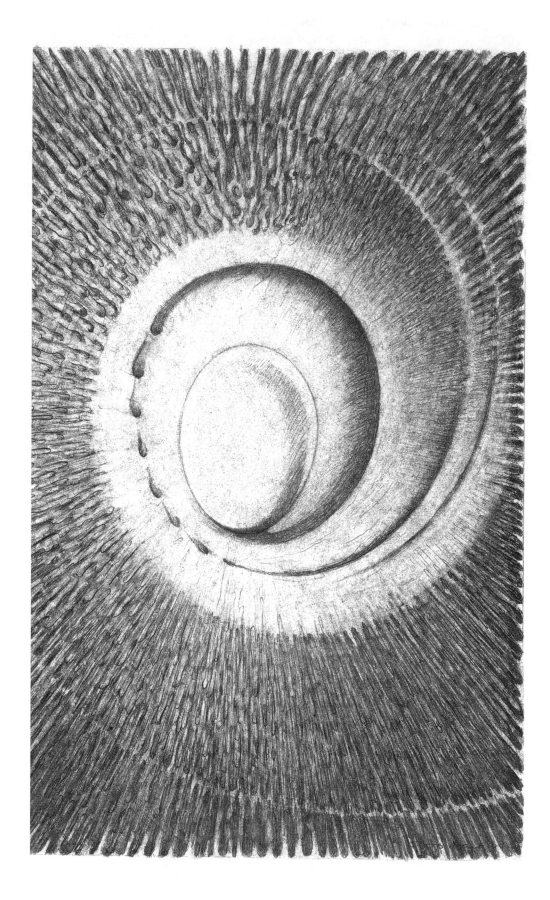

Regarding other meditations you practice
        probably they are all compatible
                as long as no harm is intended
        Just do the integration meditations
                separately from your other meditations

12. Conclusion

This edition of *Sacred Orgasms*
            is a major expansion of the previous edition
        though both focus on three tenets:
            1. We are more than a physical body
            2. Orgasms are an energetic experience
                    and sexual orgasms
                            are only one type of orgasm
            3. What we call
                    our spiritual and our sexual aspects
                        are not only
                                not in opposition,
                        they are mutually enhancing

In the future I anticipate
                at least one more book
                about orgasms
        since I close this edition
                with several questions:
        How long do we do the integration meditations
                before the ten soul centers
                        are fully developed,
                before the soul system
                        is fully developed,
                and before the soul system
                        and the seven incarnated systems
                        are fully integrated?
        What are the experiential indicators
                to know each of these three phases?
        Except for sexual orgasm,
        what do we do to easily have
                each of the other types of orgasm
                with a full intensity,
                        rather than in the very mild form
                        as in the integration meditations?

The quarter of a century of my life
                represented by these three books
                        in *The Essential Tantra*
                has been the unfolding of a mystery

The discarded "ANYWHERE" sign
            on the side of the freeway
              after my retreat at the monastery
      was a symbol of my choice
          to leap
             into the unknown
My everyday mind did not know
        where I was going
My soul just knew
        I had to go

I hope that what unfolded for me
      will have meaning for you
         should you leap
         should you feel it is time
            to dance to the beat
              of a different drum
         should you want to explore
           what is at the center
             of your sacred circle

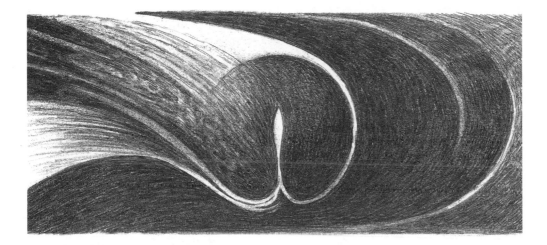

EPILOGUE

One of my principal teachers,
        a Tibetan lama,
                in response to one of my questions,
        turned to me
        and said,
                looking directly into my eyes,
    "You know,
        you already have it all
           within you."

The lama's words are also the underlying teaching of *The Essential Tantra.*

We already have it all within us: Sexuality is at the core of our existence. Without sex, we would have no body. With sex, we can touch the depths of our soul. With orgasm, we can be at-one with God.

Being of the same nature as God/Source/Goddess, our soul is far wiser, far more connected to Source than we may realize. While anyone can be a teacher reminding us, showing us how to be attentive to our inner voice, no one else is the mediator between God and us. No one else is God's emissary, delivering a set of commandments engraved in stone. Our own soul is already the mediator, the emissary.

The question, then, is how do we discover the path back to our soul—to becoming conscious of where it is all already within us.

In my quest, sexuality has taught me the most about my path. *Erotic Massage* expresses what I learned when massage became my meditation, listening to the nuances of the subtle energies. When I embraced the sexual energies, the light on my path became brighter. In *Sensual Ceremony*, bringing ceremony to the sensual-sexual dance, I found the circle, within which all becomes sacred. In *Sacred Orgasms*, I discovered the primordial beat: orgasm. And the drummer is the soul.

Living is extremely complex and trying. To say that orgasm is a sacred path to enlightenment would seem to be too simple. Many religions have laboriously laid out a labyrinth of moralities to follow in order to be allowed into heaven. To say in response to these moralities that sex is God's gift to us to find our own way back by ourselves to God would be blasphemy.

In *The Essential Tantra*, however, I am saying exactly this, that sex and orgasm are at the center of the sacred circle, that they are a catalyst to at-one-ment.

I am saying this:

When we embrace all of our sexuality,
we honor our spirituality.

When we embrace all of our spirituality,
we honor our sexuality.

When we embrace both, we celebrate God.

Sacred Sexual Positions

INTRODUCTION

Sexual positions are one of the *least* important aspects of love-making for most of us most of the time.

Yet the image of coital connection is one of the most compelling symbols for the human psyche, both in contemporary popular art and in ancient spiritual expressions.

In both Tibetan and Indian tantric sculpture and painting, a male and female secured in pelvic union is a central theme, available for all to view. The *hieros gamos,* or sacred marriage, occurred in variations in many ancient cultures. Here the king and queen or other divinely ascribed representatives would perform a coital ritual, sometimes publicly for all, often to ensure abundant fertility of crops and livestock. In the famed Indian *maithuna* tantra ceremony, partners proceed through specific, elaborate symbolic acts, including coitus, to celebrate the divine in the other, in one's self, and in all existence.

The following illustrations communicate more profoundly than the written word the meaning of sex as a sacred communion. The secret in these sexual and meditative positions is *not* how the physical bodies join. The secret is the intent the partners bring to their touch and sexual embrace. The whole being in mindfulness honors the other, without manipulation, without covert anticipations. Each moment unfolds with each partner's energies flowing freely in balance and reciprocity.

The following illustrations by Kyle Spencer appeared in the first edition of *Sacred Orgasms,* which originally was to be a book about sexual positions. When I sat down to write, though, orgasm in its diverse varieties became the central theme. I was literally living the unfoldment of the book.

Recently, I finally wrote that sexual positions book, entitled *Secret Sexual Positions,* and included Kyle's original set along with many additional illustrations of different artistic styles.

Preparing *The Essential Tantra,* I felt the initial *Sacred Orgasms* illustrations so sublimely express the natural harmony of the sexual and the sacred that I have included here the illustrations as a visual essay.

As you observe each image, take a moment to feel the presence between the two beings.

Namaste—the god within me greets the god within you—is the communion the lovers' eyes share.

This energetic communion is the sacred sexual secret.

Sex is just the beginning, not the end
But if you miss the beginning,
you will miss the end also.

Osho

Love beds are altars. People are temples
encountering temples, the holy of holies
receiving the holy of holies.

Matthew Fox,
The Coming of the Cosmic Christ

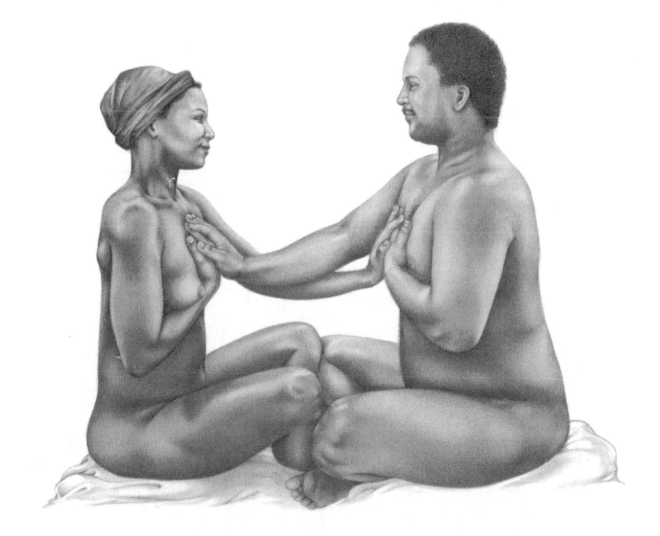

Even as fire from stone and iron springs,
From soul and body leaps the spark divine

Mahumad Shabistari, *The Secret Garden*

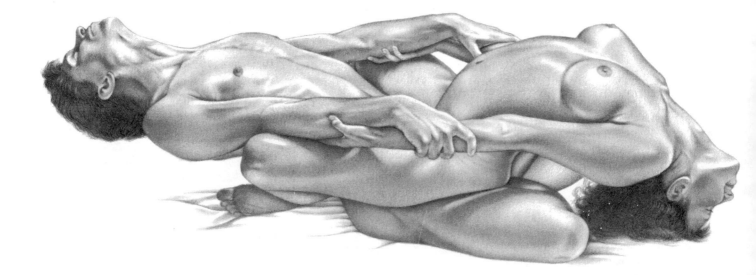

Once the Wheel of Love
has been set in motion,
there is no absolute rule.

Kama Sutra

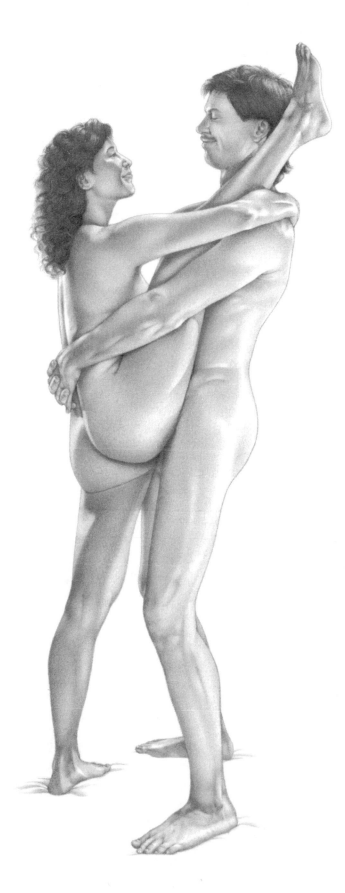

Your body is the harp of your soul,
And it is yours to bring forth sweet music
from it or confused sounds.

Kahlil Gibran, *The Prophet*

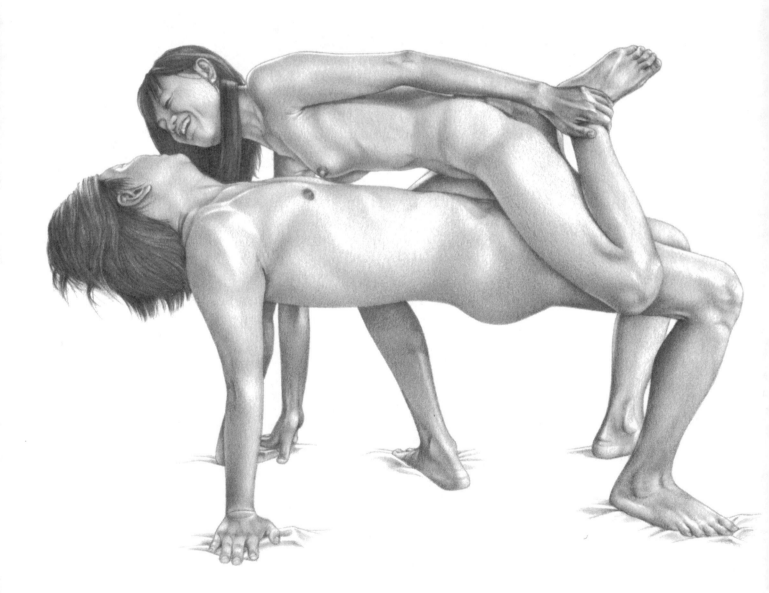

Through a tremendous outpouring of psychic energy in total devotion and worship for this other person, who is respectively god or goddess, you realize by total fusion and contact, the divine center in them. At once it bounces back to you and you discover your own.

Alan Watts, *Play to Live*

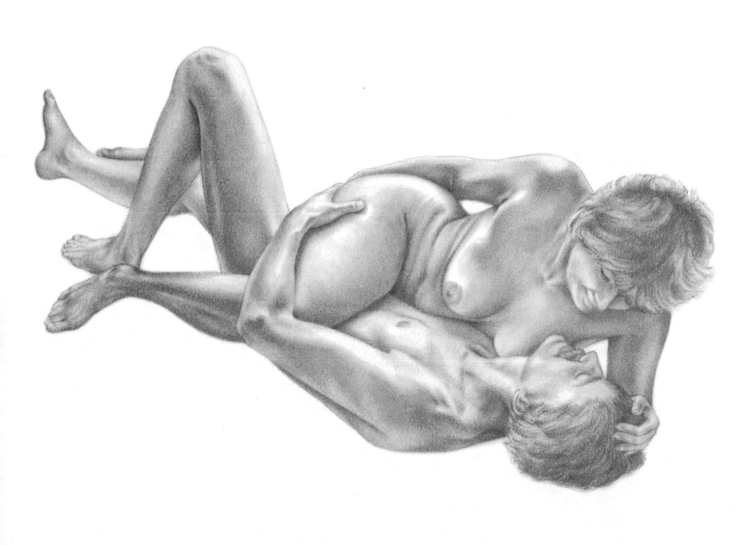

(Union is) as if in a room
there were two large windows
through which the light streamed in:
it enters in different places
but it all becomes one.

St. Teresa of Avila, *Interior Castle*

Blow upon my garden,
let its alluring perfumes pour forth

Song of Songs

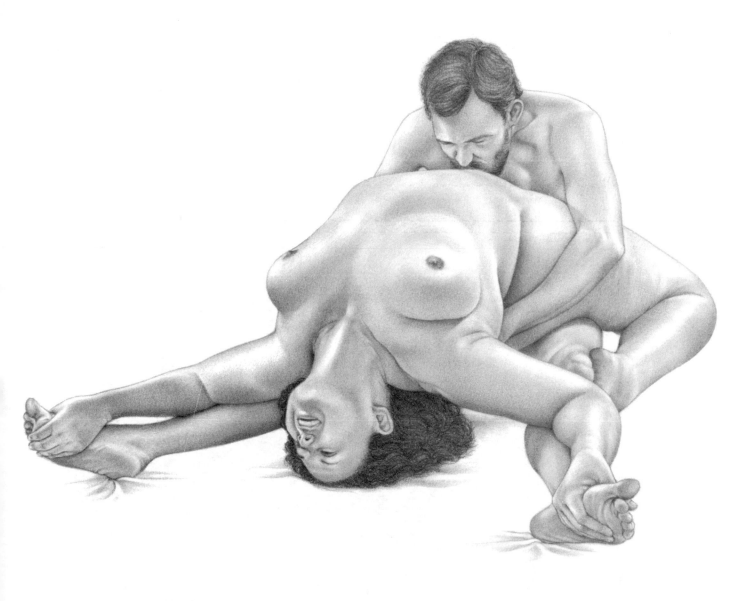

His cheeks are like beds of spice, treasures of ripe perfumes
His lips are red blossoms; they drip liquid myrrh
His arms are rods of gold
      his hands crystal olive branches . . .
His mouth is delicious, his whispers are dear,
      and his expressions, *"Desire"* itself

Song of Songs

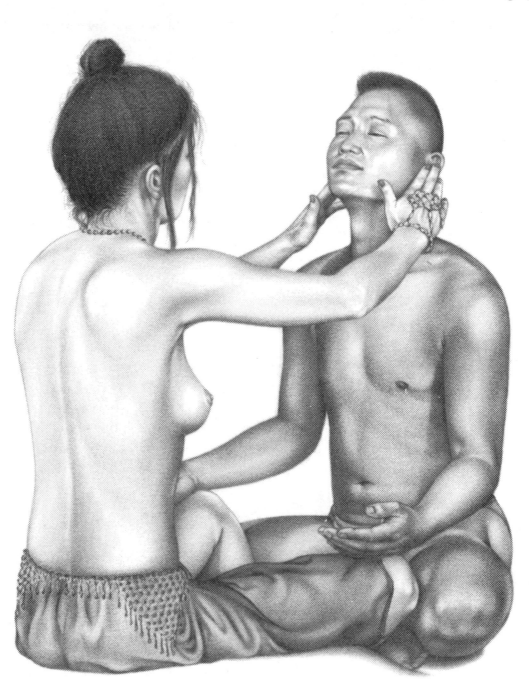

Move into the love act so deeply that the actor is no more. While loving, become love; while caressing, become the caress; while kissing, be the kiss.

Lord Shiva

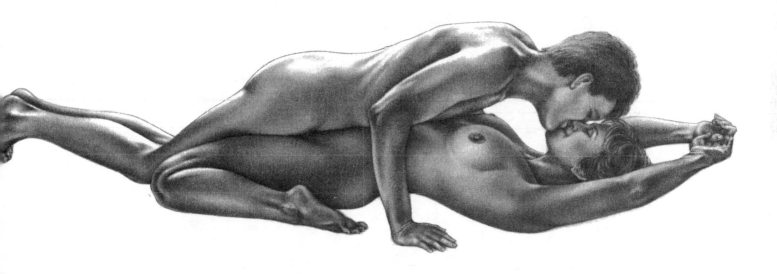

You are an enclosed garden
with a secret fountain

Song of Songs

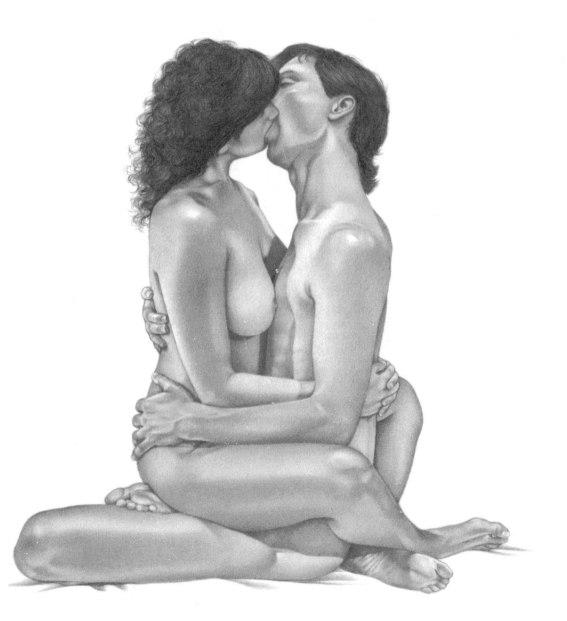

You want to travel with her
You want to travel blind
and you know that you can trust her
for she's touched your perfect body
with her mind

Leonard Cohen, *Suzanne*

My vineyard is mine to give;
my fruit is mine to give

Song of Songs

Some day, after we have mastered the winds, the waves, the tides and gravity, we shall harness for God the energies of love. Then for the second time in the history of the world, man will have discovered fire.

Teilhard de Chardin

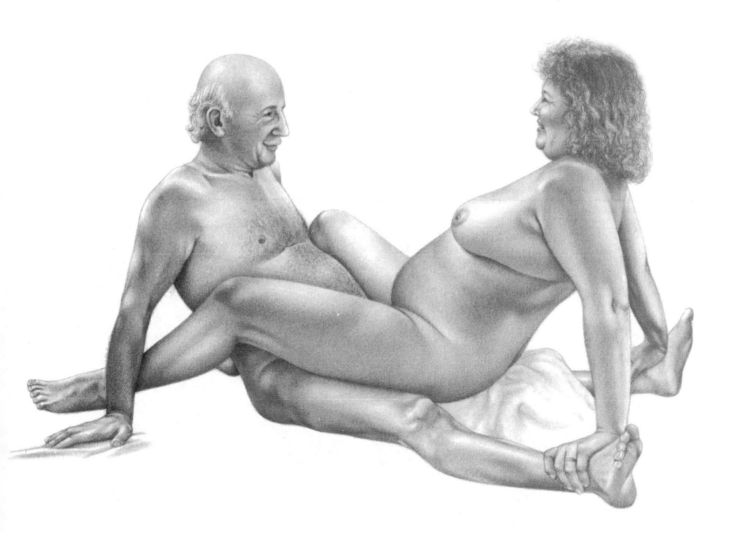

Sex has been called the original sin
—it is neither original nor sin

Osho

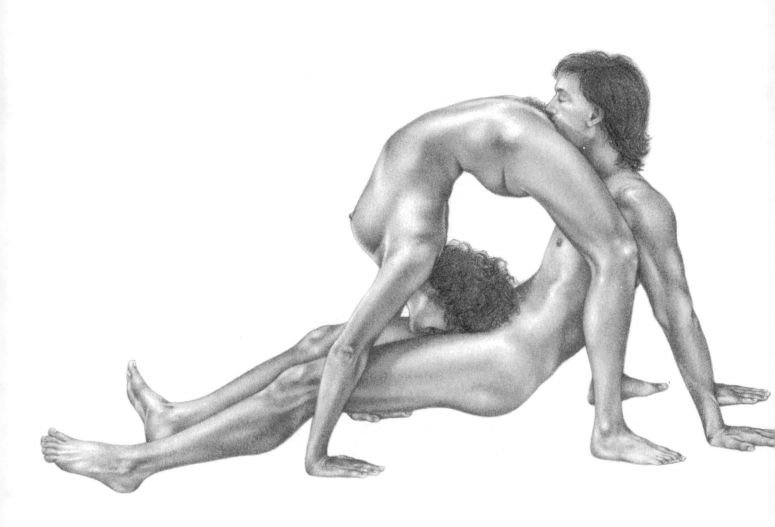

O Lord, give me chastity and continence
but not yet

St. Augustine

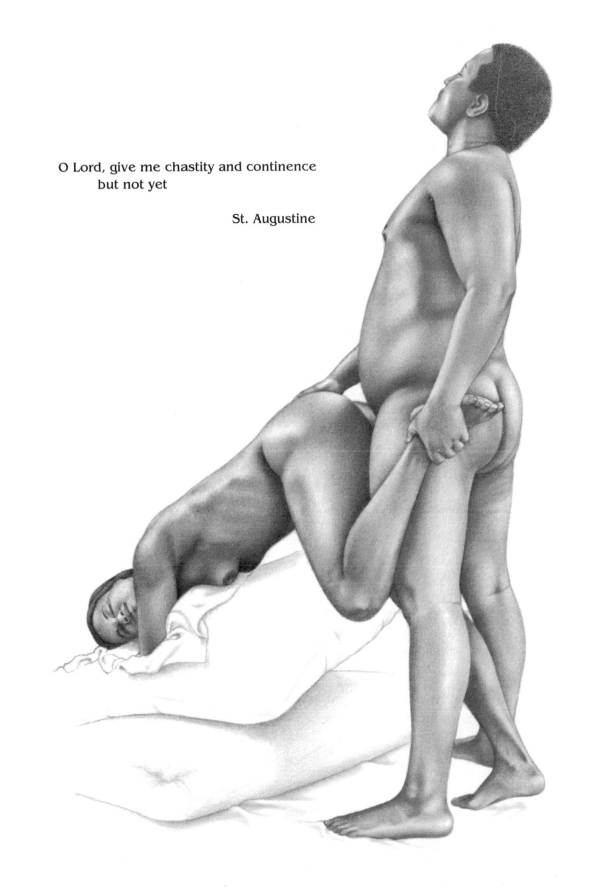

This is my body which speaks for itself .
This is my body which sings of itself

James Broughton, *Song of the Godbod*

ABOUT THE AUTHOR AND ILLUSTRATORS

KENNETH RAY STUBBS, PH.D., is both a certified masseur and a certified sexologist. He is the author of eight books and editor-contributor to *Women of the Light: The New Sacred Prostitute.*

In *The Essential Tantra,* three of his books are combined and expanded for the first time in a single volume. They reveal and summarize almost three decades of his path into spiritual traditions and both contemporary and esoteric teachings on sexuality.

Based extensively on his seminars throughout North America and Europe to both the general public and sexologists, *The Essential Tantra* is his journey of finding sexuality and orgasm at the center of the sacred circle.

He lives in the Sonoran Desert near Tucson, Arizona.

KYLE SPENCER is an artist living in Half Moon Bay, California. She graduated from the Academy of Art in San Francisco with a bachelor's degree in illustration. She is a long-time friend of the author and has illustrated a number of his books, including *Erotic Massage, Romantic Interludes, The Clitoral Kiss,* and *Secret Sexual Positions.*

Her illustrative contribution to *The Essential Tantra* include all of the art in *Tantric Massage,* diagrams one and three in *Sacred Orgasms,* and all of the art in *Sacred Sexual Positions.*

RICHARD STODART has been a professional artist for more than twenty-five years. He has received awards from the Canada Council for his painting as well as from the Pinnacle Gallery in New York for his erotic drawings. His images have been described as "sensitively thoughtful yet translucent, combining the wild electricity of wakefulness with the vivid languour of lucid dreaming."

His works appear in magazines and as book covers and illustrations. He has exhibited his paintings and drawings in Toronto, the San Francisco Bay Area, New York, Vermont, Virginia, and Hawaii. A native of Trinidad in the West Indies, he is a Canadian citizen currently living in the U.S. He can be contacted at 512 Old Glebe Point Road, Burgess, VA 22432.

In *The Essential Tantra* he contributed all the illustrations in *Sensual Ceremony,* and *Sacred Orgasms* with the exception of diagrams one and three.